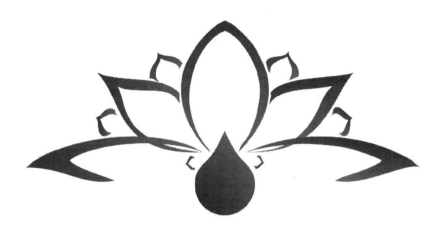

ESSENTIAL YOGA PRACTICE

Your Guide to the New Yoga Experience with Essential Oils

MONA FLYNN, MS, E–RYT 500 • ASTI ATKINSON

This book is dedicated to my family: to my husband who gives me space and time to pursue the dreams that call me, to my children without whom I would not have energy and inspiration, and to my mother who always reminds me that I can do anything.

Mona Flynn

To my boys, Benjamin and Joshua, who inspired the partner sequence of this book so the new yogi in me could learn to connect with them on an even deeper level, to my husband who supports all my ventures and continues to teach me that everything is okay, to my closest friends who show me unconditional love, and to all those who are ready to embark on their own personal journey of growth in body, mind and spirit.

Asti Atkinson

ISBN-10: 1514626187
ISBN-13: 9781514626184
Library of Congress Control Number: 2015910017
CreateSpace Independent Publishing Platform
North Charleston, South Carolina

FOREWORD

When I began teaching yoga in 1981, only a select portion of the population was interested in the practice. Today yoga has become very widespread reaching into every segment of our population.

In more than three decades of teaching, I have had the pleasure of introducing many to the practice of yoga, as well as training and inspiring many a yoga teacher.

When Mona came to study with me, she was green around the edges and in need of healing. By the time she graduated from my 500-Hour Transformation Yoga Teacher Training Program, the light of wisdom had been lit, and she emerged as a valuable teacher in her own right.

I am pleased to acknowledge that Mona has continued to study and refine her skills, as you will see reflected in the pages of this book.

In my experience, the healing journey is essentially the same for all of us. We come face-to-face with our fears, embrace our confusion and uncertainty, pray for guidance, and commit to those practices that will help us on our journey. Learning from a teacher who has taken the healing path to heart offers the greatest value to the student. Mona is clearly one of those teachers.

If you have been fortunate enough for this book to have landed in your hands, you will find a welcoming outline introducing you to yoga. The yoga sequences offered will support you on your healing journey and help you build the sensitivity needed to make better choices for balance in your life.

You will also become part of an evolutionary journey that combines the use of essential oils and yoga as self-help tools on the healing path.

It will be of great interest to see how this combination of natural healing remedies unfolds as each individual person shares his or her experience. Such a unique opportunity can be found inside these pages.

May you find healing, peace, and happiness.

Lillah Schwartz
Nationally recognized master yoga teacher and adaptive yoga and back care specialist. Author of *Healing Our Backs with Yoga*™, *A Layman's Guide to Back Pain Relief* and two therapeutic DVDs—*Yoga: Your Freedom from Back Pain* and *Yoga: Relief from Neck and Shoulder Pain.*

ACKNOWLEDGMENTS

As this is our first book and DVD, we learned quite a lot about the process of writing, editing, publishing, social media marketing, and videography. The professional and technical folks involved were patient and helped educate us with regard to understanding both the process and the product's goal. We have stuck to our initial goal for this book: to present the accessibility of a yoga practice to students of varying ages, sizes, levels of fitness, and histories of practice—from seasoned students to novices. We wanted to show everyday people enjoying and building resilience with the practice of yoga enhanced by the use of essential oils.

At first we anticipated the need to perform everything on our left side while cueing the viewer for the right side. Though this ended up being a mistake, we chose not to redo the videography as the original participation of the students was sincere, their practice reflected our intention, and their volunteer time was valuable. In turn this presented an incredible editing challenge, but we think the viewer might enjoy the captivating and encouraging practice of these true yogis.

In each sequence the viewer gets to see that yoga is a "practice" because we are not perfect. This gives permission to the new student—the viewer—to begin to learn without judgment. No matter how seasoned a student, we want to arrive each time at our practice with the eyes of a beginner, and learn something new, both about ourselves as well as the process.

As we are planning the next book with more DVD sequences, we will continue to follow our goal of offering variety in a yoga asana practice. We will combine introducing and building with the other limbs of yoga while still allowing anyone to begin to participate and experience personal growth through yoga and essential oils on all levels—body, mind, and spirit. Our efforts, our attention and our intention reflect how we take the lessons of our yoga practice "off the mat," applying what we have learned and being open to continuing to learn along the way. As the joy is in the journey, we continue to learn with one another.

We hereby acknowledge the following people and organizations for their contributions to this project; please see a complete listing at the back of the book:

Sam Hamlin and Joy Hardy of Technical Event Management, for their willingness to listen to the endless detail of editing requests and also for their videography.

Christ United Methodist Church, Greensboro Performing Arts, and Stillwaters Retreat, for the use of their facilities for our photography and videography.

All the individuals who filmed with us, for their willingness to practice and record yoga sequences and for their time given generously to this project.

Ariel Seymour, Matilda-Kirby Smith, Cassie Shintay, Marci Trakas, Sam McClenaghan, and Lauren McSwain for their work on the photography and cover designs.

And of course, we must acknowledge our spouses and children. They supported us through endless conference calls, editing sessions, and writing time, and they participated in a number of critical activities behind the scenes. Thank you all for your love and support!

Mona Flynn and Asti Atkinson

PREFACE

Yoga is the perfect opportunity to be curious about who you are.
—Jason Crandell

By Mona Flynn:
The foundation of our yoga journey is self-discovery on all levels: spiritual, emotional, and physical. With this in mind, we designed this book *Essential Yoga Practice* to be a great starting place if yoga is new to you and perhaps a great place to Agrow if you are a seasoned student as we are marrying two practices for which we have a great passion: yoga and essential oils. Both practices will help you along the journey to self-understanding and self-discovery in all three areas—body, mind, and spirit—not only complementing each other, but perhaps also creating an exponential value when practiced together.

Though yoga came to us long ago from the East—from India—the practice has traveled well through time, past the age of Sanskrit as an everyday language, into the present, and well into the West. Slowly, we are recognizing the importance of bringing our yoga practice back to its roots, especially because of the challenges of everyday modern life. Considering this ideal intention, we not only hear the term *yoga practice*, but also *yoga therapy*. We begin to widen our scope of practice to all eight limbs of yoga, as well as to apply the study of yoga's sister science, Ayurveda, also a five-thousand-year-old practice, which is where we find some direction on the use of essential oils.

As a young exercise physiologist fresh out of graduate school, my interest and outlook was to use my academic knowledge as a tool to "fix" mechanical issues in the body. One particular challenge at the hospital where I worked was an assignment to lead classes for people with severe osteoporosis and rheumatoid arthritis. After getting to know the participants in the classes and applying what I knew then, I felt that I had only a short list of "safe" movements for them to practice and felt challenged to find more. That is how I came to study yoga. I bought many books and was thrilled to discover more than just *asana*—the physical practice—and soon recognized the need to have a formal teacher. Two decades later, I have watched many people come in the door for both private and group yoga classes, studied with many well-established teachers, and started my own yoga business, and co-founded a yoga school. Though I now work to certify teachers, I still want to help provide a safe starting place for whoever is new to joining us on this journey.

Yoga teachers and studios are set up for group classes in the West, teaching mostly asana and pranayama (breath work). Group classes are recognized as a means for students to learn how to practice in order to build their own growing personal practice. Studios begin to teach students to honor many of the limbs of yoga practice by removing shoes, phones, and chemical influences such as perfumes or heavy scented lotions and deodorants. Yoga students also honor the practice by being timely and orderly, putting away props, and showing respect to one another and to the teacher. Many yoga teachers and studios do not yet know enough about the use of essential oils—especially pure oils—to recognize where and when to begin to incorporate them. In this book, we hope to educate and inspire more yoga teachers to implement their use skillfully for the benefit of all their students. After all, as we are all teachers, we should not teach what we do not know.

My first experience with yoga in combination with essential oils was in 2002 when I attended a yoga training session. The teacher introduced an essential oil blend to use for fatigued and stressed muscles. It was quite effective and opened my eyes to the potential use of essential oils. Immediately, my mind realized the emotional benefits because the aroma of this blend was also quite reviving. I came away from that weekend teachers' training looking for how to begin studying the use of essential oils. I found many books, and after scouring through them, I looked for various companies from which to purchase essential oils. I kept coming up against the disappointing realization that most of the products had fillers and incorporated the use of synthetics. For that reason, I did not share using oils with my family nor in my classes other than the original blend that my teacher shared. Purity—for the sake of safety—was important to me.

It was not until I discovered essential oils that I found to be consistently pure and potent that I felt confident sharing oils that were safe for my family and students. I began to put a couple of drops (mostly of citrus essential oils) in a pitcher of water outside the classroom. I incorporated arriving to class early to run a diffuser for group classes. I educated my students on usage of essential oils and offered a drop in the palm of their hands either at the beginning of a practice or at the end—just before a restorative pose. My students loved learning and using the essential oils, and we have continued to learn together. If I forget to offer an oil at the beginning of our practice, now they remind me. This has added immensely to our journey of self-discovery and practice of yoga overall, sparking the interest to delve into the other limbs of yoga practice.

We live in a harried, hurried world where we are overwhelmed by being overly connected to other people and to information systems. This adds to our stress levels immensely on a daily basis and begins to affect our energy, posture, digestion, immune system, sleep patterns, and general outlook. We seek to nourish ourselves on a spiritual and emotional level as well as on a physical level. We seek the opportunity to learn how to have clarity and a sense of peace. Carving out some time for self-care can lead us in that direction. Using yoga comprehensively and learning how to use essential oils are both great tools, and here is where time and experience make the difference.

As we travel through the four stages of life, we see ourselves change and grow with the life lessons and hurdles that crop up daily. There is the time of initial awakening into adulthood. This is followed by early young adult life where we come into fullness finding our place in this world to use our gifts and begin to make our mark. There is midlife to early old age where we find ourselves more comfortable with speaking our truth and then old age where our wisdom comes more from the heart, based on life experiences. In all of these times, we find common threads of daily rituals for self-discovery and self-care and using what is natural allows us to connect more to our true nature, to other people, and to our world. We learn many things from and with one another along the way. We stumble in places, and we reach out to help pull one another up as well. We learn and relearn, fine-tuning our awareness.

Luck is what happens when preparation meets opportunity.
—Lucius Annaeus Seneca

Both yoga and essential oils can be used daily to support physical well-being, to improve spirit, bring peace of mind, boost energy, and provide clarity for making choices that resonate with one's intuition and grounding. How and what we choose to use may differ from one person to another as we are all such unique individuals. After all, it is called a "practice."

After I spent three years using essential oils in my own yoga practice and with my students, I traveled to an international educational conference on essential oils. During the conference, I met with Asti Atkinson. That meeting resulted in combining our knowledge and experience to educate yoga teachers and studio owners in a way to introduce the use of all-natural essential oils to group practice sessions.

Combining our knowledge and experience, we wanted to begin to educate yoga teachers and studio owners that it is acceptable and beneficial to introduce the use of all-natural pure essential oils to group practice sessions. Most studios ask that students do not use perfume and strongly scented cosmetic and toiletry items when in class. This is because some people will have an adverse reaction to the aroma of such products, which are made with synthetics. However, when using *pure* essential oils aromatically to calm, energize, uplift, relieve stress, breathe more deeply—or to clean mats/ the yoga room—the added value to the group yoga class experience will provide an additional opportunity for personal growth and a myriad of health benefits. It is an opportunity for the yoga teacher/ yoga therapist to educate students on the use of more than just asana practice. Ideally, students come to group practice to learn how to build their home practices. Truly, this is an additional opportunity for teachers to guide students on the practical use of aromatherapy for themselves and their families in everyday life.

In this book, we will share with you some of what we have learned. You will find a brief introduction to yoga and its history. You will also find an overview on essential oils that introduces history, science, and common uses—and you will become aware (if you aren't already) that all essential oils are *not* created equally.

Each friend represents a world in us, a world possibly not born until they arrive, and it is only by this meeting that a new world is born.
—Anaïs Nin

by Asti Atkinson:

I discovered essential oils in 1998 when a friend shared some of them with me. That was the first time I had considered natural alternatives to support health and wellness, and I was intrigued with the possibilities. I quickly discovered that all essential oils were not consistent in quality. I experienced firsthand the importance that sourcing, harvesting, extraction, and testing have on the purity and potency of the end product.

I remember the first time I tried a peppermint essential oil that truly resonated with me. I put a drop on my hands, rubbed my hands together, cupped my nose, and inhaled. Because I had a few bottles of peppermint essential oil at home already, I wasn't prepared for the power and purity that I experienced in that moment. In a microsecond, I felt invigorated and my breathing felt clearer. I was hooked! I learned that *pure* essential oils have the ability to support the healthy function of our body systems...and then my excitement grew.

My passion for using and sharing natural solutions for health and wellness led me to become a wellness advocate and educator in 2010. I loved teaching others how to incorporate pure essential oils into their lifestyles to assist with their emotional and physical well-being.

I met Mona at one of those classes, which led to my interest in yoga in connection with the application of pure essential oils. A friend and I scheduled a private yoga session with Mona, and I was surprised and astounded at the depth of the experience Mona facilitated for me in this session. Immediately, I recognized I was working with a true master of her art. Mona was someone who understood the body and the spirit, had dedicated herself to training and learning, and knew instinctively how to coordinate a complete yoga experience to promote healing and connection on an incredibly intimate level. I felt myself connecting not only to my own spirit and feelings, but also to the space and people around me. I can only describe it as completely beautiful and awe inspiring.

Since that time, I have never passed up an opportunity to work with Mona. My respect and admiration for her knows no bounds, and I know I am one of many that she has touched. She is well respected in both her geographical community and in the yoga community. I am excited for the birth of her new yoga school (Institute of Integrated Yoga Therapy) to train instructors in traditional and cutting-edge methods of mind-body practices including Tension and Trauma Releasing Exercise (TRE), Pilates, and Ayurveda.

I am also excited and grateful for the opportunity to collaborate on this important project with Mona. In our conversations, we came to the realization that many people had experience with either yoga or essential oils, but not in combination with each other. So, we set out to create a book that provided a foundational education on yoga and essential oils as well as how to use them together to enhance the benefits of each. The book was written in such a way that both new and advanced oil users—as well as new yoga students and advanced yogis—will benefit from the information.

Mona has choreographed six original yoga sequences with carefully selected themes designed to produce powerful results. New yogis may not recognize that the safety, benefits, and overall experience provided by each yoga sequence is attributed directly to the talent, insights, knowledge, and prior yoga training of its creator. This means Mona's incredible yoga training with experienced yoga instructors, together with her Master's degree in Exercise Physiology—combined with her twenty years of teaching yoga—have resulted in these simple yet profound sequences. Add to that the targeted use of pure and potent essential oils, and prepare yourself to experience yoga like you have never done before—this is *Essential* Yoga Practice.

Yoga is the journey of the self, through the self, to the self.
—Bhagavad Gita

We hope that you will enjoy and benefit from this book as much as we have benefited. The book and DVD were created from the heart, and we hope you will recognize the treasure that is found within this program.

ABOUT ESSENTIAL YOGA PRACTICE

Personal yoga practice builds individual self-awareness and an understanding of our strengths, desires, and place in the community. It also enhances our awareness of where we are in the present moment, and perhaps even our clarity of where we are going. Our time on the mat is contemplative and results in lessons that serve our growth "off the mat" as well. For example, when we build time in any pose, we quickly find that staying even a little bit longer presents us with a quickly increasing amount of work physically, with regard to strength, flexibility, balance, stability, and this leads to emotional challenges. Certain emotions may arise and we learn by noticing our reactive habits: How might we respond to an unexpected challenge on the mat? Does this represent our typical response to challenges off the mat? In this case, what do we do when things become difficult?

While the majority of the book can serve as an excellent resource, the section you will come back to again and again is the collection of Iyengar-influenced Hatha yoga sequences that bring awareness to the breath and add value to the movement during transitions.

Seasoned students grow to realize that with building time in each pose, there is opportunity for building self-awareness. Self-awareness is also built through the transitions to each successive pose, which in turn provides a space for building mindfulness. Through it all, the intentional focus on the breath brings opportunity for transformation.

The sequences are designed to be user-friendly, whether you wish to use the book or the DVD to follow along. Through repeated practice of these sequences, you will grow in many ways. You will become stronger in body, mind, and spirit.

You will find the following sequences in this book:

Morning sequence:

- Provides grounding and energy
- Contributes to an awareness of where you are starting so you can have clarity, direction, and energy for where it is you're going

Strengthening sequence:

- Recharges both the body and the mind

Detox sequence:

- Creates space between vertebrae
- Establishes space and relief in body and mind
- Helps you let go of what is unnecessary
- Infuses your organ systems and body frame with more nourishment and energy

Partner sequence:

- Encourages you to connect on a deeper level with your partner or child
- Allows you to recognize and experience the value of your connections to others as well as the healing capacity that traction offers

Sleep Easy:

- Provides release from unnecessary worry
- Quiets both mind and body

Restorative Practice:

- Helps you recognize how to support the body so that muscles relax
- Encourages deep rest so the body can heal and restore optimal health

It is our desire that you use and enjoy this book for your personal growth and well-being. For additional tips and updates, please visit our Essential Yoga Practice blog (www.EssentialYogaPractice.com) regularly.

Enjoy your journey!

Namaste!

TABLE OF CONTENTS

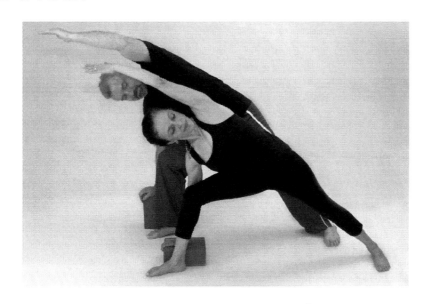

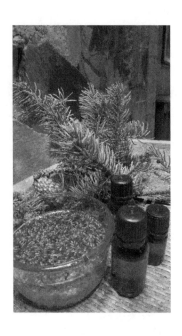

Section 2: Ayurveda - The Sister Science of Yoga · · · · · 13

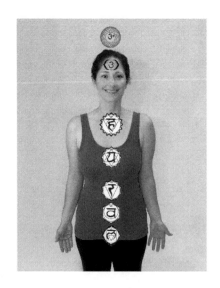

Section 3: The Chakras - Energy Centers of the Body · · 27

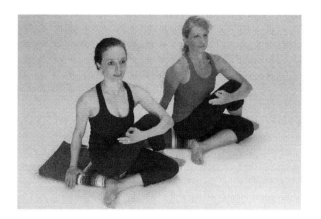

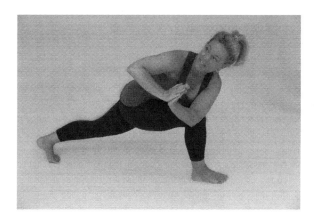

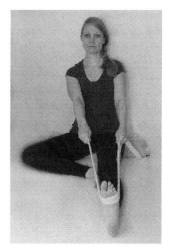

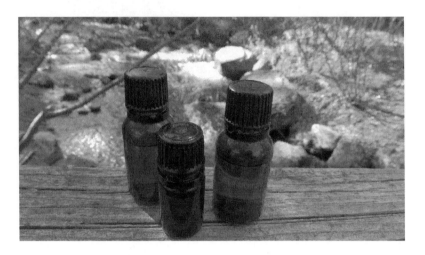

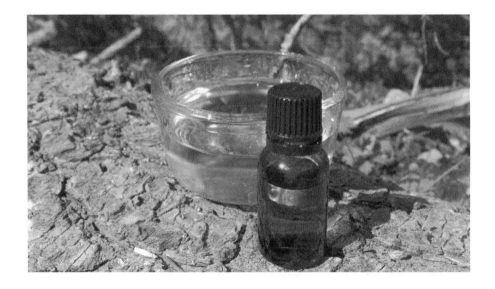

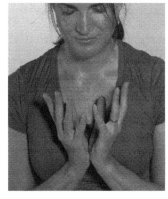
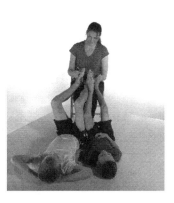
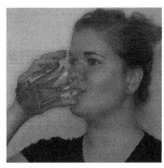

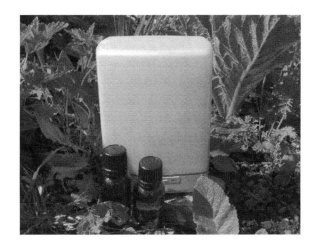

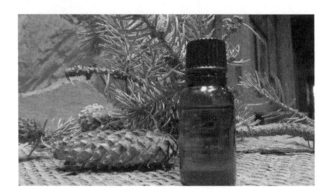

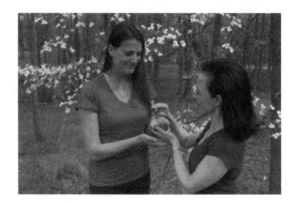

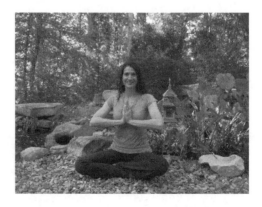

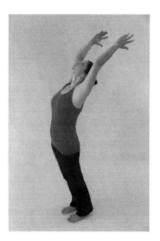
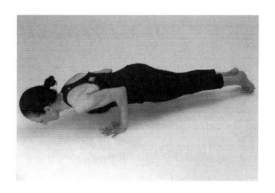
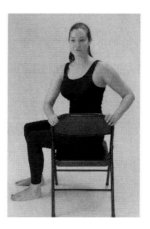

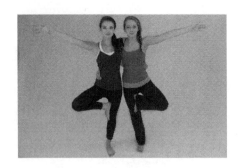

Sequence 4: Mom/Dad and Me (Partner) Sequence ·· 161

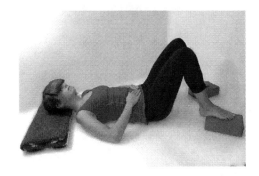

Sequence 5: Sleep Easy Sequence · · · · · · · · · · · · · · · · 177

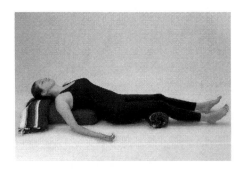

Sequence 6: Restorative Poses · · · · · · · · · · · · · · · · · 193

PART 1: YOGA

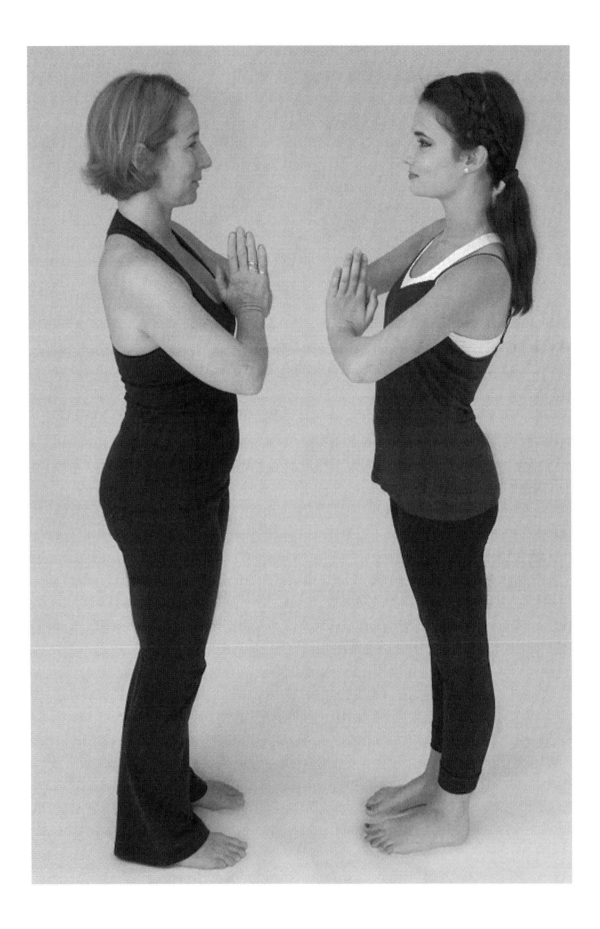

SECTION 1: INTRODUCTION TO YOGA

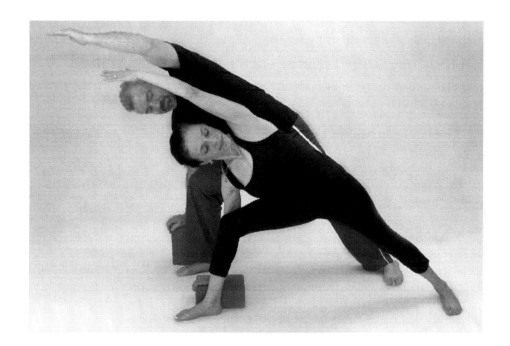

Yoga, an ancient but perfect science, deals with the evolution of humanity. This evolution includes all aspects of one's being, from bodily health to self-realization. Yoga means union—the union of body with consciousness and consciousness with the soul. Yoga cultivates the ways of maintaining a balanced attitude in day to day life and endows skill in the performance of one's actions." —B. K. S. Iyengar

Yoga is a buzz word these days, and people interested in it are coming to the practice for many reasons: to improve their fitness, to release tension, to slow down, in order to create balance in their lives on a daily basis. The word, *yoga*, in Sanskrit means to "yoke" or "bind"; the union here is between body, mind, and spirit. These are the three aspects about our lives that we must attend to in order to learn more about ourselves and to grow.

Yoga came to us from the East—from India—and has persevered for about five thousand years, evolving over time. It is a comprehensive practice that incorporates much more than what we consider as yoga in the West. We recognize the physical practice and look to participate in group classes, read books, and watch DVDs to learn what and how to practice at home.

Probably the most famous of all yoga philosophers was Patanjali, who was considered to be the father of yoga as he documented the yoga sutras in the second century BC. Until then (and still), the eight limbs of yoga through the sutras were passed down orally from teacher/guru to student. The sutras are 195 verses/aphorisms on how to live life in order to achieve enlightenment. They describe the Eight Limbs of Yoga, known as ashtanga yoga. Following this classical eight-limbed path will free us from physical, emotional, and mental suffering. This is a tried-and-true path that has equivalent guidelines in almost all the faith disciplines. So, despite initial doubts, newcomers to yoga find that the practice will allow them to be more grounded in their own faiths.

Yoga teaches us to cure what need not be endured and endure what cannot be cured.
—B. K. S. Iyengar

The Eight Limbs of Yoga outlined by Patanjali comprise a nonreligious guide that outlines how to live with good intentions, while seeking personal growth and transformation. Discipline, self-study, and surrender to God are the cornerstones of the sutras, which also point out that the biggest mistake we make in our life journey is to think we are separate from God. This echoes many faith practices as well. If we were to look at guidelines for proper living in all faith practices, we would find all of these ideals are outlined in a similar way.

As yoga came to us from India, the language at the time was Sanskrit and to this day, students all over the world use Sanskrit terms as they study and practice. Interestingly, if you were to travel and decide to take a group asana class, you would find it possible to follow based on the fact that a well-educated teacher would use the Sanskrit terms to introduce the poses of the sequence.

1. Yamas (Restraints)

There are many definitions of ahimsa and to parallel one of the Ten Commandments, "Thou shalt not kill," is a straightforward understanding of the word. On a deeper level, ahimsa guides us to living with more compassion and to curbing the immediate rash reactions that come from anger. Ahimsa also stresses that we must not mistreat ourselves—we must honor the body as a temple, and take care of ourselves on all levels.

Forgiveness, love and our connection with the Divine is the medicine that is healing the sickness of our time."
—J. Artos Roske

a. Satya—Truthfulness

Again, all faith practices include direction that means, "Thou shalt not lie," so we connect easily to this yama. However, here we are encouraged to speak the truth even when it is easier to do nothing in a situation, or when it is easier to hide behind something that masks the truth. Also, we must be thoughtful with how we use our words and combine them with good intentions.

Wisdom is found only in truth."
—Johann Wolfgang von Goethe

b. Astea—Non-stealing

Here, we understand we must not take what is not ours, nor covet what others have. This extends to the success of others, not just to material objects. Recognizing our individual gifts helps us to be who we are meant to be. Desiring what we lack causes suffering. We want to strive to be comfortable with what we have and who we are in order to feel stable and happy. Our work is to discover our gifts and use them.

Be thankful for what you have; you'll end up having more. If you concentrate on what you don't have, you will never have enough.
—Oprah Winfrey

c. Brahmacharya—Abstinence

> *All the gold which is under or upon the earth is not enough to give in exchange for virtue."*
> —Plato

Much is written/translated in this yama. Patanjali may have meant celibacy with the idea that sexual energy takes away from the ability to focus on devotion. In our modern day, the idea is not to use your sexuality in a reckless way. You will be respecting yourself as well as others.

d. Apiragraha—Non-greed

> *Travel light, live light, spread the light, be the light.*
> —Yogi Bhajan

In our modern world, we are exposed to a lot of things. Nonattachment to material goods becomes a lesson to be learned by all of us. In learning nonattachment, we learn not to associate happiness with tangible items. On a broader scale, we learn to recognize the many blessings in our lives and not just the material things we have and need, but health, family, relationships, faith...our list of blessings is endless. Perhaps then, we might not long for what is unattainable.

2. Niyamas (Disciplines)
a. Saucha—cleanliness

> *Honor the physical temple that houses you by eating healthfully, exercising, listening to your body's needs, and treating it with dignity and love.*
> —Dr. Wayne Dyer

Saucha here means much more that being clean in your living environment. It means being pure in your thoughts and in what you consume—not just what you eat but also what you use on your body. Taking care of the body as the temple, being truthful, and consuming pure products are all a part of saucha.

b. Santosa—contentment

> *Yesterday is gone. Tomorrow has not yet come. We have only today. Let us begin.*
> —Mother Teresa

This might be considered the ultimate rule—to live in the present moment. Our harried and worried thinking, our long lists of things to do, fear and anger that we don't deal with, our obsession in planning for our future...all of these things overshadow the many opportunities of the present moment, which come from what we learn from awareness.

c. Tapas—Austerity

The Sanskrit word, *tap*, means "to burn," so "tapas" means "heat" from the perspective of discipline. Practicing tapas is what helps us to get up on time, to apply our efforts to whatever needs consistent attention (like our yoga asana practice), and to show up for life rather than to shirk responsibility or take the easy way out. It also drives us to stand up for what we believe and for how we were raised.

d. Svadhyaya—Self-study

The practice of svadhyaya dictates that the better you know yourself, the more likely you are to have control over your actions, your thoughts, and your emotions. Living mindfully helps you to be a more responsible participant in all the ways you are connected to your world—your family, friends, church, school, country, and to your Higher Power.

e. Isvara Pranidhana—Devotion to God

Patanjali never cited a particular deity figure in the sutras. Instead, we are encouraged to dedicate our devotion to our Higher Power. Our world is filled with many faith practices. Hopefully, we will not see our differences, but instead, how much more we are alike. Most faith practices are very similar in dictating how to live with good intentions, how to honor others around us and ourselves, and how to include religious study to align closer to our Higher Power.

> *Self-discipline begins with the mastery of your thoughts. If you don't control what you think, you can't control what you do. Simply, self-discipline enables you to think first and act afterward.*
> —Napoleon Hill

> *Unless you learn to face your own shadows, you will continue to see them in others, because the world outside you is only a reflection of the world inside you.*
> —Author unknown

> *Truth is one. Paths are many.*
> —Swami Satchidananda

3. Asana (Physical Practice)

Yoga is the dance between the light and the dark within you. The light is what brings you back to the mat and the darkness is what you uncover there. Don't be afraid of this darkness; these are only shadows and though you'll have to walk down some pretty dark alleys, remember you are grounded in the light and that light will set you free."
—Amy Jirsa

The physical practice of yoga is the "asana" practice—the "poses." Just as there are many poses, there are many preparations for poses. All of these are very comprehensive building blocks. You should strive to practice all of the various kinds of poses—standing, seated, reclined, twists, inversions, and restoratives. The various angles of holding the body against gravity will strengthen the health of the spine with respect to *extension*, which maintains the space between each vertebra to allow discs and nerves to perform effectively.

Learning to build time holding a pose yields more than just the strength certain muscles need to hold that pose. You will learn the balance of actions within the alignment of your frame to provide safe progress with regard to strength and flexibility. You will cultivate stillness that allows connection to body and breath and makes peace with the fluctuations of the body to hold on to the work of the pose as well as the mind, to maintain its focus. Most importantly, you will build awareness to learn the emotional and spiritual lessons of each pose.

Building time in each pose allows self-study and the release of stagnant and stuck energy in the chakras. The ultimate goal of an asana practice is to strengthen the body so as to allow you to tolerate sitting for long periods in meditation. This fine-tunes your ability to focus on the meditation instead of straying toward the habit of fluctuating thoughts. Ultimately, this paves the way for the journey toward enlightenment.

When you inhale, you are taking the strength from God. When you exhale, it represents the service you are giving to the world.
—B. K. S. Iyengar

4. Pranayama (Breath Work)

Prana is energy and *ayama* means control. Breath is the life force and our focus on our breath—specifically on slowing down our breath—has many advantages. It calms the central nervous system, puts things in perspective, counters the physical effects of stress, builds lung capacity, increases mobility of the rib cage and diaphragm, and lays the foundation for the following limbs.

Meditation is a way for nourishing and blossoming the divinity within you.
—Amit Ray

5. Pratyahara (Mind-withdrawal)

In our overly connected world, pratyahara is quite useful in helping us pull away from external stimuli and returning to what is necessary right in front of us. With inward withdrawal, we get to fine-tune our awareness of our personal needs, as well as our surroundings without being overwhelmed and ruled by them.

Concentration can be cultivated. One can learn to exercise will power, discipline one's body and train one's mind.
—Anil Ambani

6. Dharana (Concentration)

Intense concentration is required for meditation. It is the foundation and is cultivated in all of the previously mentioned yamas and niyamas.

7. Dhyana (Meditation)

The thing about meditation is: You become more and more you.
—David Lynch

Meditation is the real "game changer" in yoga practice. A daily meditation practice is very effective to countering stress, directing a change of perspective, and perhaps even to providing clarity, as the mind gets a break from both daily chaos and mind chatter. It is the key to building awareness and to the ultimate aim of yoga—enlightenment.

The goal of life is to make your heartbeat match the beat of the universe, to match your nature with Nature.
—Joseph Campbell

8. Samadhi (Enlightenment)

Samadhi is the product of the cultivated practice of all the yamas and niyamas. Here we have a great balance in how we live life and, more importantly, how we are not shaken by anything. Our actions and intentions become pure and solid. We live with ease and feel as if we are one with everyone and our universe.

The Five Sheaths

A comprehensive and consistent yoga practice yields a positive impact on anything that has to do with body function as well as emotional and spiritual well-being. Yoga works to create this harmony by removing blockages in all areas. Yoga practice will help you build your awareness about how you function—also on many levels. As our primary attention goes to the body, we learn about our five layers, the five koshas, known as the five sheaths. When we practice yoga—asana, pranayama, meditation, mantra and karma, we have an effect on one or more of these layers.

- **Annamaya kosha** is the outside layer of the body, the physical body. It is made of our bones, muscles, tendons.
- **Pranamaya kosha** is the energy body and *prana*, or energy, moves around the body through the *nadies*, or channels—there are seventy-two thousand. Asana practice affects these first two koshas. Over time and practice, blockages are worked through and the regained flow of the body's energy will result in better overall health.
- **Manomaya kosha** is the mental body. Most people are attracted to yoga to benefit the first two koshas. However, they stay with their regular yoga practice because of how it affects mental clarity positively, and intuitive nature that revolves around safety and emotional needs.
- **Vijnanamaya kosha** is the deeper level of internal wisdom and the sense of higher knowledge and building this awareness takes dedicated practice. We tap into compassion, love, and joy here.
- **Anandamaya kosha** is the bliss body, where the yoga taps deeper to reach enlightenment, realizing that he/she is one with the all that is—especially with God.

As yoga practice deepens, and blockages are released, it is not unusual to have spontaneous release of emotion. This is an opportunity to let go of what holds you back in life. So, if the emotions are connected to a sadness or anger, it is the yoga practice that is helping to release them in a nonharmful way by opening your body, mind, and spirit to recovery and true well-being.

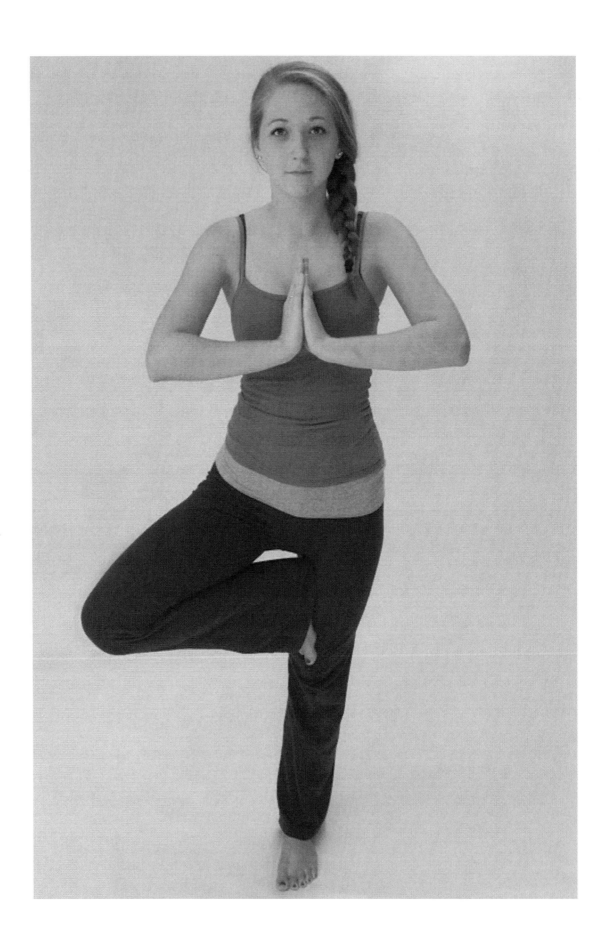

SECTION 2: AYURVEDA – THE SISTER SCIENCE OF YOGA

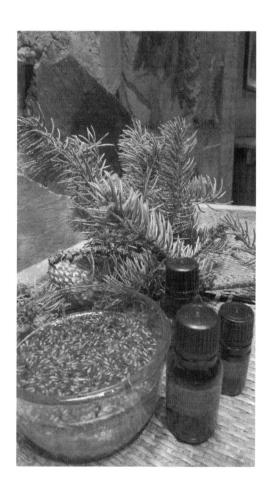

Your lifestyle—how you live, eat, emote, and think—determines your health. To prevent disease, you may have to change how you live. —Brian Carter

Ayurveda translates from Sanskrit to the "knowledge of life." Like its sister science, yoga, it dates back five thousand years to the ancient texts—the *Vedas*. Like yoga, it is a system of healing and is considered the "medicinal arm" of yoga. Ayurveda looks at our physical constitution, emotional nature, and spiritual outlook with regard to or place in the universe. In each of us, the universal life force manifests as three different energies, constitutions, or "doshas:" vata, pitta, and kapha.

Each of us is made up of our own unique combination of these doshas. This unique combination is determined at the moment of conception and is called your "prakruti." At the end of this section is a table used to help you assess your unique prakruti, with your predominate dosha(s). Some people tend to be dominant in one, yet almost everyone is dominant in two doshas. Your prakruti does change as you move through different stages of life and it can fluctuate with the change of the season, environment, diet, age, climate, and other external factors. The effect that these external factors has on your doshas can cause doshic imbalance—*vikruti*. In turn, this will affect energy, many aspects of health, and mood.

Everything is made up of five elements: Air, ether, earth, fire and water. Each dosha is affected by one or more of these elements, which in turn affects bodily functions, emotional well-being and spiritual outlook. In your yogic journey to discover yourself, learning with regard to your own constitution will offer you a greater sense of body awareness— especially with regard to more personalized preventative health practices and more specific healing practices unique to your constitution. Ninety-five percent of attention in Ayurvedic medicine is spent on the preventative side of the practice, so primarily think about your prakruti to establish your healthy lifestyle practices.

When our system is challenged, or out of balance, we must then think about vikruti with the ideal of pacifying the dosha that is the most prevalent in the imbalanced state. In addition, seasonally, your outlook to pacify potential doshic imbalance can be easily effective, following seasonal principles of Ayurveda. For example, in the summer, follow the Pitta program; in the fall, follow the vata program; in the winter, combine vata and kapha programs; and in the spring, it is time to focus more on vata management. These principles vary depending on where you live and how each season expresses the elements and qualities associated with the dosha.[1]

Vata—The Energy of Movement

Vata is influenced by the air and ether elements. Vata dosha predominates all bodily movement in the form of sensory stimuli and motor responses. Vata-dominant people are quick to think and move, very creative, flexible, learn quickly yet forget easily. They are alert, restless, active, yet fatigue easily. Mentally, they volunteer, initiate, participate in conversation, yet often speak without thinking. Physically, they are lean with dry skin. They have curly coarse hair, cold hands and feet, irregular digestion with a tendency for bloating and constipation, and their sleep habits are light and irregular. Prone to worry when there is an imbalance, they can obsess over making wrong decisions and become convulsive and erratic.

Vata is more prominent in the fall and early winter, so it is key to be careful of diet and routine at this time of year. Vata-dominant people respond more to warm, moist, and heavy foods with warming spices, steam baths, humidifiers, daily abhyanga practice, and body massage with significant oils high in the emollient factors—such as almond, coconut, and olive oils.

Like the air, it is hard for vatas to become grounded, so yoga poses that activate the pelvis, hip, and thigh are key—such as the following:

- Uttanasana (Standing Forward Bend)
- Vrksasana (Tree)
- Virabhadrasana II (Warrior II)
- Gomukhasana (traditional Cow Face pose from sitting with knees stacked)

---

1 Dr. Vasant Lad and Maria Garre, *Ayuroga*, The Ayurvedic Press (2014) Print

- Salamba Sarvangasana (Shoulder stand)
- Bhujangasana (Cobra)
- Ustrasana (Camel)
- Baddha Konasana (Bound Angle pose)
- Ardha Matysendrasana (Half Lord of the Fishes)
- Virasana (Hero)
- Pawanmuktasana (Wind Releasing pose)
- Surya Namaskar (Sun Salute) with a slow steady rhythm focusing on deep breathing

Take care of your body. It's the only place you have to live. —Jim Rohn.

Prayanama for vatas should include choices that build the inhalation as their tendency is to have a much easier exhalation. Agni Sara, Anuloma Viloma, Bhramari, Kapababhati, Nadi Shodhana, Utgeet, and Ujjayi are good options.

Pitta—The Energy of Transformation

Pitta is influenced by both fire and water elements. Pittas are generally strong physically with a medium build. They are intense and easily irritable. Their skin freckles and reddens easily with exposure to sun, massage, heat and strong emotion. They are strong willed, stubborn, stand up for what they believe is right, work and play with intense competitiveness. Pittas think and learn quickly while being impatient with others who are less focused. Pittas have high metabolism and strong digestion.

Pittas are natural leaders with great planning abilities, and they seek material prosperity. They tend to have acid indigestion and loose stools. Pittas prefer hot spices and cold drinks, yet they need to balance their fieriness with sweet, bitter, and astringent tastes. Their blood sugar drops easily, and they are especially grumpy when hungry. They need to balance their high-energy lifestyle with rest—for both body and mind—and include a consistent and significant meditation practice.

Their abhyanga practice is best with coconut and sunflower oils. Pranayama for pittas includes Agni Sara, Chandra Bedhana, Kapalabhati, Sheetali, and Sheetkari. Since pittas typically lead an intense, fast-paced lifestyle, grounding and centering practice is a great way to stay focused and keeps pittas from depleting their energy. Yoga asanas for pittas include the following:

- Utthita Trikonasana (Triangle pose)
- Parivritta Trikonasana (Revolved Triangle pose)
- Ardha Matysendrasana (Half Lord of the Fishes)
- Setu Bandhasana (Low Bridge pose)
- Bhujangasana (Cobra)
- Dhanurasana (Bow)
- Matsyasana (Fish pose)
- Navasana (Boat)
- Supta Virasana (Reclined Hero pose)
- Balasana (Child's pose)
- Chandra Namaskar (Moon Salute) with attention to navel and solar plexus

Kapha—The Energy of Lubrication

Kapha is influenced by water and earth elements. People who are predominantly kapha have a strong frame. They are naturally athletic as long as they are exercising regularly; otherwise, they gain weight very easily.

They are calm, tolerant, forgiving, and have high endurance in every way so that they are seen to be stable, compassionate, and loyal. Kaphas are very methodical, prefer regular routines, and do well professionally for these reasons. Naturally, they seek to balance themselves with interest for new environments, people, foods, and life experiences.

When out of balance, kaphas become unmotivated, stubborn, and depressed. Usually, they are attracted to sweet, salty, and oily foods and need to balance them with bitter, astringent, and pungent foods and tastes.

Their sluggish metabolism makes kaphas gain weight easily, be less interested in exercise and be more prone to colds, flu, mucous buildup/congestion, edema, diabetes, water retention, and congestive headaches.

Kapha-balancing diets are more important during winter and early spring. The diets should avoid beef, heavy dairy, iced food and drinks, fatty, oily, and fried foods. Regular physical activity is especially necessary to invigorate both body and mind. In addition, kaphas should avoid napping during the day.

Abhanga practice with corn, mustard, and sesame oil is best. Pranayama practice for kaphas includes Agni Sara, Bhastrika, Brahamri, and Kpalabhati. Asana practice for kaphas includes the following:

- Parsvottanasana (Pyramid Pose)
- Virbhadrasana II (Warrior II)
- Utthita Parsvakonasana (Side Angle Pose)
- Urdhva Hastasana (Volcano Pose)
- Nataranjasana (King Dancer pose)
- Salabhasana (Locust pose)
- Urdhva Dhanurasana (Wheel/backbend)
- Urdhva Prasarita Padasana
- Simhasana (Lion pose)
- Surya Namaskar practiced vigorously being mindful to open chest and shoulders

Use the following Dosha Assessment to see where you align. Select the trait under each category that most applies to you. Note that (V) responses correspond to vata, (P) to pitta, and (K) to kapha. When you are finished, calculate your results to discover your dominant constitution(s). Add totals to determine your personal constitution or dosha(s). Note that most people are bi-doshic, meaning that they are dominant in more than one type.

Dosha Assessment

Trait	Vata	Pitta	Kapha
Face Shape V P K	oval thin chin long Neck	angular, square moderate chin, jaw medium neck	round face and chin short neck
Teeth V P K	crooked, small, grey	medium, yellow	large, white, straight
Eyes V P K	small, dark, darting, active	medium, deep set, intense sensitive to light	large, gentle, moist light color, thick lashes
Nose V P K	small, uneven, deviated septum thin bridge	pointed, red, medium size	large, round, wide bridge
Lips V P K	dry, chapped, pale, thin	medium, red/pink	full, smooth
Hair V P K	dry, brittle, brown, curly/wavy, unruly	straight, blonde/red, balding, early gray, oily, fine	coarse, thick, lustrous, oily, wavy
Skin V P K	thin, dry, rough, wrinkles, cold, tans easily	medium, fair, slightly oily, moles, freckles, burns easily	thick, soft, moist, pale, smooth, tans slowly/evenly
Nails V P K	dry, rough, brittle	medium, flexible, healthy nail beds	thick, hard, smooth
Musculature V P K	long thin muscles, bone structure visible	moderate, firm	moderate to large muscles, develop quickly
Frame/Bones V P K	thin frame	medium frame	broad/stocky frame
Belly V P K	thin/long	moderate	big, round
Appetite V P K	variable, forgets to eat, prone to low blood sugar crash	moderate to strong, always hungry	low appetite, steady blood sugar, doesn't like to skip a meal but handles it well
Digestion V P K	bloating, forms gas	good, quick digestion, prone to heartburn	slow, heavy, mucus-forming
Elimination V P K	irregular, constipation	normal to loose, once or more daily	large, sluggish once daily
Weight V P K	doesn't gain weight easily	easy to lose extra gained weight	gains weight easily, loses slowly
Subtotals:			

Trait	Vata	Pitta	Kapha
Body Temperature V P K	always cold, especially hands & feet, barely sweats	mostly warm, good cirulation, sweats easily	adapts easily to varied temperatures, tends to feel cool, reliable
Moods V P K	changes moods easily, changes mind easily	opinionated, ready to express opinions	stubborn, steady, slow to change, yet reliable
Task Completion V P K	likes to start tasks, has difficulty finishing	starts and finishes tasks, cares about completion	happy to work on tasks but lets others initiate
Organization V P K	disorganized, scattered	very organized	cluttered, keeps sentimental objects
Memory V P K	good short term memory, poor long term memory	good short term memory, especially with daily tasks	distinct, specific, convenient long term memory
Sleep V P K	sleeps lightly, awakens easily	sleeps soundly, awakes refreshed	sleeps late, naps when possible
Stress Habits V P K	often worried, anxious, overwhelmed	often frustrated, impatient, irritable, but focuses on tasks	avoids difficult situations, withdraws and shuts down
Personality Traits V P K	enthusiastic, lively, hyperactive, anxious, leader, spontaneous	driven, competitive, jealous, problem solver, strategic	loyal, grounded, nurturing, compassionate, sentimental, reliable
Decision Making V P K	difficulty in making decisions, changes mind constantly	makes decisions easily, often in haste	slow to decide, makes decisions carefully
Mental Energy V P K	creative, active mind, scattered thoughts	organized thoughts, pays attention to detail	doesn't like to be rushed, steady thought process, sometimes foggy
Physical Energy V P K	varied tendency toward hyperactivity, crashes	moderate to intense	slow, lethargic
Speech Patterns V P K	speaks quickly with enthusiasm	speaks clearly and concisely	speaks deliberately, thoughtfuly
Subtotal:			
Totals Table 1 & 2:			

Summary
Though our constitution is determined at the time of conception, as one passes through the seasons of life, the seasons of the year, and experiences certain emotional and physical setbacks, the dominance of certain doshas will change. As our dominance shifts from what is our true constitution, this may present as "dis-ease" in the body, and may also affect emotional and/or spiritual well-being. Sometimes, this dosha imbalance is evident to us and with learned awareness and self-study, we can attend to imbalances before they get out of hand.

In the practice of Ayurveda, health is considered order and disease is disorder. From the cellular level, to the body's system, and even an integrated level of the entire body, there is constant interaction between order and disorder. Our internal environment is in a constant flux and is reacting, as well, to our external environment.

Because we can find order and understanding within disorder, we can use self-study, experience, and discipline to return to order. Furthermore, in Ayurveda, the understanding of health is necessary to building body awareness so that when there is a change or shift from optimal health, we can have a reference point. Therefore, as you perform your personal dosha assessment, focus on the answer that represents you during the majority of your healthy life, not necessarily your current condition. Individualized Ayurvedic practices, with this reference point are the foundation to maintaining wellness.

According to Dr. Vasant Lad, an internationally established Ayurvedic doctor and author of many text books on ayurveda, "dis" means "deprived of" and "ease" means "comfort." Before discussing disease, we must understand the meaning of comfort and health. A state of health exists when the digestive fire (agni) is not stagnant, the bodily humors (doshas) are in equilibrium, the three waste products (urine, feces, and sweat) are produced at normal levels and are balanced, the senses are functioning normally, and the body, mind and consciousness are working harmoniously."[2]

This balance is responsible for both natural resistance and immunity. The person who has this balance is quite resilient to disease, even contagious disease. Imbalances in body and mind are responsible for disease. Looking at the bigger picture of health and disease, the practice of Ayurveda addresses physical, emotional, and spiritual health. The use of essential oils supports healthy function in all three of these areas.

Ayurvedic Massage

In Ayurveda, the daily routine of self-care—dinacharya—includes abhyanga, or massage. Large amounts of warmed carrier oils are used in abhyanga. Herbs and essential oils are commonly added to the carrier oils. Massage can be received from a massage therapist or done personally in the morning and should take about 15 to 20 minutes.

There are several types of massage—full body, face, abdominal, and foot massage. Ayurvedic massage is very holistic. It is used preventatively to help with elimination of toxins as well as to help create balance in the body to aid in overall wellness.

Ayurvedic massage takes into account the dosha, the nadis (pranic currents of energy in the body), the 107 energy points (*marmas*), the three gunas (subtle mental temperaments responsible for behavioral patterns), and the seven dhatus (tissues of the body). Abhyanga is followed by Sweda karma—a sweating process such as in a sauna—to help with further elimination of toxins. When done at home this can be a hot shower, a warm bath, or consist of wrapping the body with warm cloths.

Another technique is Shirodhara in which warm oil is drizzled on the forehead at the third eye for 30 minutes to aid brain function and induce feelings of calm, which is often a precursor to a sense of rejuvenation. While on a massage table wrapped in warm towels, the warm oil—sometimes infused with fragrant essential oils—flows in a slow, steady stream over the scalp and through the hair. This helps to stimulate the endocrine system, the pituitary and pineal gland, and the pleasure neurotransmitter. The process also helps to synchronize alpha brain waves, aid circulation to the brain, improve mental clarity, and release deeply trapped *ama*, or toxins.

Ayurveda dictates that routine play an important role in health. A healthy life is one dedicated to recognizing and supporting one's prakruti, or unique constitution. It is better to have a daily routine that defines daily actions such as the waking time according to one's body clock followed by a morning cleansing routine and then meditation. Thus, certain abhyangas are to be done in the morning—such as body or abdominal massage—and certain abhyangas are used more before retiring in the evening, such as face and foot massage.

A carrier oil is used in abhyanga to moisten the skin and support the seven dhatus. The dhatus are part of our biological protective mechanisms and with the help of agni, or digestive fire. The dhatus are responsible for the health of the immune system of the body.

Oiling the body will first excite the excess dosha by loosening it and the sweda process helps to sweat it out. It is ideal to be in a pure state when you do abhyanga, thus it is recommended as part of the morning ritual. Typically, the carrier oil is warmed. All the qualities of oil are exactly opposite the qualities of vata (dry, light, rough), and in Ayurvedic practice, it is said that 80 percent of physical or mental imbalances are vata based.

Vata-dosha governs the nervous system so abhyanga will soothe, calm, and nurture vata—especially when you do not rush abhyanga. Because vata-dosha is very dry, oil will help moisten vata attributes. Pitta is sharp, so the softness of the oil will help pacify pitta imbalances. Kapha tends to be dull, and the oil will offer richness.

Interestingly, different carrier oils can add a beneficial layer to targeted doshas. For example, sweet almond oil is used for pitta-dosha.

Coconut oil is also good for pitta, but it depends on the person and on the climate. It is not recommended in the winter or in cold environments. Pitta dosha individuals can also use safflower and sunflower carrier oils. Kapha dosha individuals benefit from using mustard oil, flax, organic corn oil, and olive oil.

For additional targeted dosha support, pure essential oils can be added to the massage oil carrier. For vata dosha, use an essential oil that is sweet, earthy, and warming such as any citrus oil, lavender, Roman chamomile, and/or vetiver. Pittas are hot, so they need cooling oils such as sandalwood, rose, geranium, Roman chamomile, melaleuca, and frankincense. Kaphas need stimulating oils such as spruce, eucalyptus, white fir, ginger, and rosemary.

There are specific regimens to help support healthy body functions such as digestive wellness—in Ayurveda we use almond or sesame carrier oil and peppermint, cardamom and/or ginger essential oil(s). Also available are the herb-blend and carrier-oil combinations that come from recipes dating back several thousand years. For example, mahanorayan oil, which has over eighty different oils and/or herbs and is cooked/prepared in a specific way, supports muscles and joints.

Snahana means "to oil" and also means "love." When we give an oil massage—an abhyanga massage—we are giving it with love to help body, mind, and spirit.

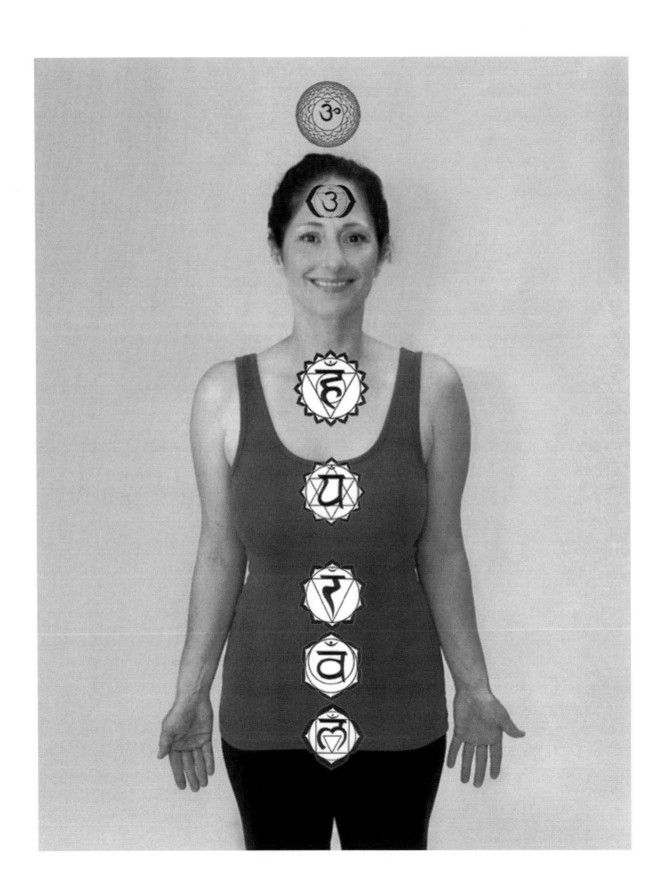

SECTION 3: THE CHAKRAS – ENERGY CENTERS OF THE BODY

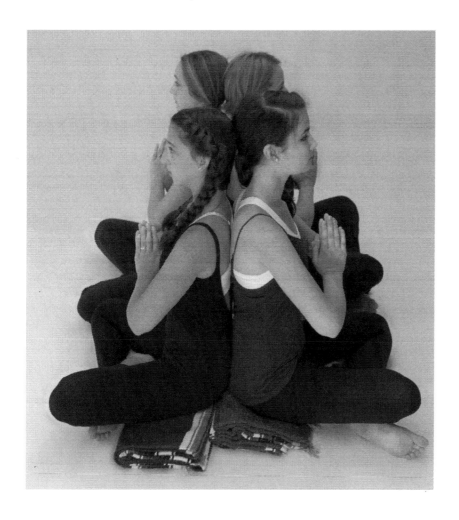

The body never lies. —Martha Graham

There are seven major energy centers located along the spine. Each of these seven *chakras* represent a different part of one's identity and is influenced by physical, emotional, and spiritual health. Each chakra is located along the *shushumna nadi*, or central breath channel, and is associated with a major plexus of nerve, artery, and vein meridians.

What is occurring in each chakra can equally influence different aspects of physical, emotional, and spiritual health.

The Sanskrit word, "chakra," means "spinning wheel." The energy of our chakras is always spinning clockwise, and if we perform fluid, turning movements—as in the practice of the Five Tibetans in yoga—we always turn clockwise to avoid getting "stuck" in a certain chakra. Physical issues begin to manifest when there is obstruction in any of these energy centers and imbalance can occur—being either excessive or deficient—instead of the healthy, freely flowing energy between the chakras that we want to maintain.

To support healthy balance, there are many avenues of approach. Ayurvedic medicine, diet, meditation, affirmations, vibrational healing of certain stones; practicing specific yoga asanas, mudras, breathing techniques, vibrational sound healing therapies; and of course, the use of essential oils are all examples.

To learn about and understand the requirements of maintaining balance in the chakra system, we will recognize the opportunity of acting on the side of prevention in being wellness advocates. When we are born, we live mostly in our lower three chakras, Mulahadra, Svadhishthana and Manipura. As we mature and take our place in our world community, we "grow up" into the ascending chakras as our true life journey is toward our connection to our Higher Power.

As you study the chakra chart, look to each category as you consider the importance of using various yogic practices in order to enhance the vitality of your chakras. This is useful especially if you are experiencing the need for attention to a certain chakra. As you become familiar with the relevance of each category and as you learn through the experience of the use of the "tools" available—such as mantra, yoga asana, essential oils, color, stone, meditation, and so on—the bigger picture will unfold. Your intuition will guide you as to what you may need to practice to help with resilience in a certain chakra. Thus, with time and practice, you will begin to understand yourself a little more. You will find effective ways to decipher the physical and emotional messages as well as address the nurturing of each energy center.

Yoga is not just repetition of few postures—it is more about the exploration and discovery of the subtle energies of life.
—Amit Ray

When we learn and spend time in yoga practice and open our chakras so we're not stuck emotionally and/or physically in any single chakra, we are better able to harness the energy and intelligence of the higher three chakras—Vishudda, Ajna and Sahasrara—and bring them to the heart chakra, the Anahata. We are also better able to harness the energy and intelligence of the lower three chakras—Mulahadra, Svadhishthana and Manipura—and likewise bring them to the heart chakra. Then we lead with the heart.

Name	Color / Symbol	Location	Element	Mantra	Significance	Body Part(s)
Mulahadra	Red	Root or Base Chakra	Earth	LAM	Grounding, Survival, Security Heritage	Legs, Spine, Adrenal Glands
Svadhishthana	Orange	Sacral Chakra	Water	VAM	Creativity, Sexuality, Sensuality, Vitality	Reproductive Area
Manipura	Yellow	Solar Plexus Chakra	Fire	RAM	Power Center, Self-will, Individuality, Self-esteem	Digestive System
Anahata	Green	Heart	Air	YAM	Pure Love	Lungs
Vishuddha	Blue	Throat	Ether	HAM	Clear Communication	Throat, Ear
Ajna	Purple	3rd Eye	Mind	OM	Clear Vision	Eyes
Sahasrara	White	Crown	Spirit	OM	Inspiration Bliss, Connection to Higher Power	Central Nervous System

Name	Yoga Identity	Yoga asana	Essential Oil	Stone	Meditation
Mulahadra	Physical Identity	Uttanasana (standing forward folds), Janu Sirsasana (head to knee pose)	Bergamot, Vetiver, Cinnamon, Ginger, Myrrh, Patchouli	Bloodstone, Tiger's Eye, Black Onyx	Meditate on one's connectedness to others and of one's importance in the many circles one is involved in; this will boost self-confidence.
Svadhishthana	Emotional Identity	Trikonasana (Triangle), Eka Pada Rajkapotasana (Half King Pigeon), Baddha Konasana (Bound Angle Pose)	Sandalwood, Orange, Geranium, Cedarwood, Jasmine	Garnet, Ruby, Carmelian, Amber	Meditate on happiness, creativity and passion.
Manipura	Ego Identity	Ardha Matysendrasana (Half Lord of the Fishes), Tadasana (Mountain), Navasana (Boat)	Juniper, Lemon, Neroli, Peppermint	Amber, Moonstone, Sunstone, Tiger's Eye, Ametrine	Focus on one's inner light and opportunities to radiate that inner light.
Anahata	Social Identity	Bhujangasana (Cobra), Ustrasana (Camel), Garudasana (Eagle)	Bergamot Ylang Ylang	Rose, Amazonite, Green Jasper, Jade, Rose Quartz, Tourmaline, Turquoise	Meditate on leading with the heart, the true center of intuition
Vishuddha	Creative Identity	Salamba Sarvangasana (Shoulder Stand), Simhasana (Lion), Halasana (Plow), Ustrasana (Camel).	Geranium, Bayberry, Chamomile, Myrrh	Blue Adventurine, Blue Agate, Blue Jasper, Lapis, Turquoise	Focus on feeling fully alive, releasing suppressed feelings, and speaking one's truth.
Ajna	Archetypal Identity	Anjanyesana (Low Lunge Crescent), Sirsasana (Headstand),m Balasana (Child)	Lavender, Camphor	Purple Adventurine, Amethyst, Orange Adventurine, White Jade, Flourite, Lapis Lazuli	Meditate on guidance from inner wisdom.
Sahasrara	Universal Identity	Vrksasana (Tree Pose), Padmasana (Lotus)	Frankincense, Lavender	Amethyst, Crystal Quartz, White Agate, Opalite, Howlite, Selenite, Sapphire	Meditate on honoring the body as the temple of the radiant soul.

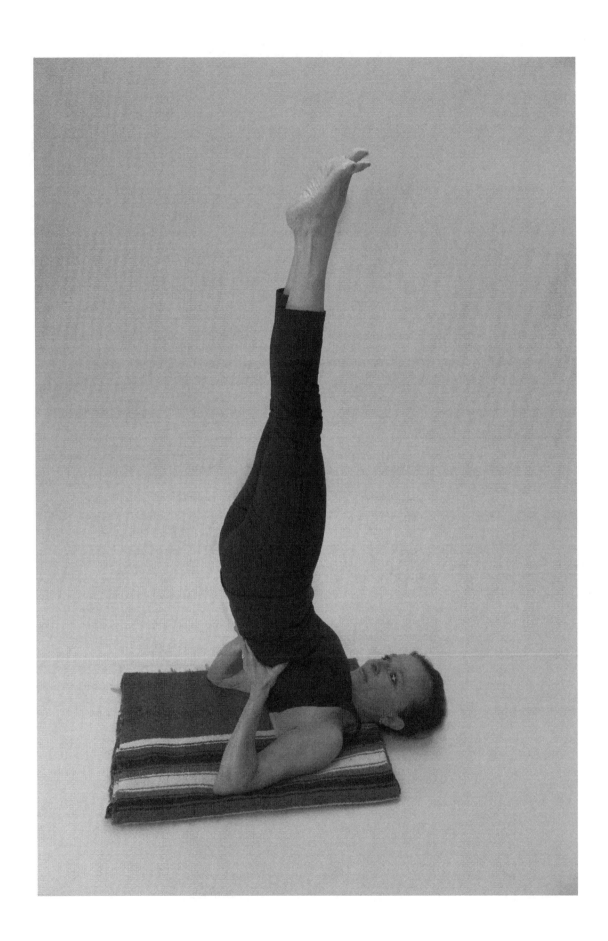

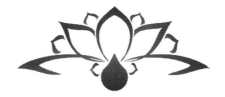

SECTION 4: BENEFITS OF YOGA

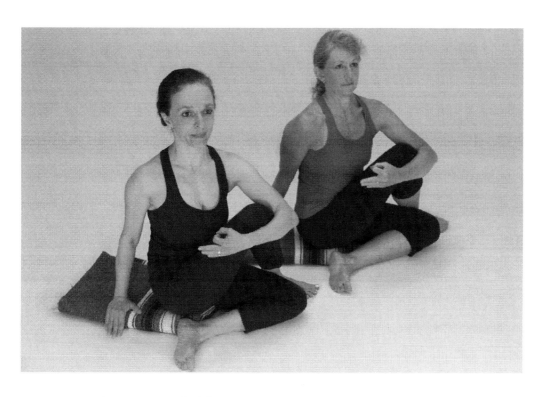

For those wounded by civilization, yoga is the most healing salve. —T. Guillemets

The benefits of a consistent yoga practice are many, and rather impressive. The growing use of yoga in the West is in the area of yoga therapy—an interesting return of using not just asana but also the other limbs of the practice to meet the individual student's unique needs. Therefore, yoga therapy is being used like physical therapy, yet more comprehensively. Keeping this in mind, yoga has a place for people with physical limitations. It is a great tool in sports medicine as well as occupational and psychological therapy.

Yoga asana practice improves the following:[2]

- Overall health and well-being
- Components of physical fitness—flexibility, muscular strength, muscular endurance, cardiovascular endurance, and balance
- Allergies
- Body Awareness
- Body Mechanics in Daily Movement
- Bone strength
- Cellular renewal
- Chronic Disorders
- Circulation
- Concentration
- Digestion
- Emotional Health
- Energy level
- General Positive Outlook
- Headaches
- Immune Function
- Lung Capacity
- Lymphatic Health
- Mobility
- Mood management
- Occasional Strains
- Pain management
- Posture
- Relaxation
- Self-Acceptance
- Sleep
- Spiritual Health
- Stress management
- Weight management

---

2 Dr. Tim McCall, MD, *Yoga as Medicine*, (New York, New York, Bantam Dell, a Division of Random House, 2007), 47.

Yoga may help to reduce the following:

- Necessary amount of medication
- Stress and tension, both physical and psychological
- Back injury/issues
- Blood pressure
- Depression
- Fatigue
- Inflammation
- Negative outlook on life

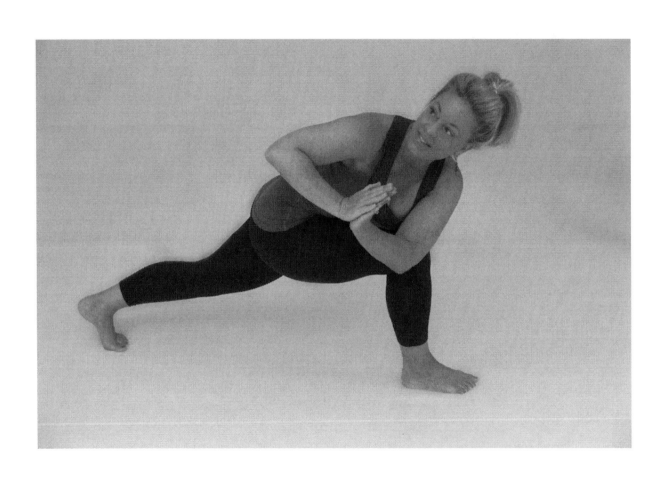

SECTION 5: HOW YOGA MAKES YOU FIT

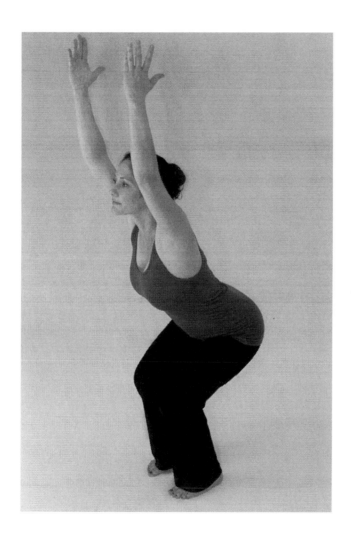

Do your practice and all is coming. —Sri K Patthabi Jois

What defines overall "fitness?" Most dictionary definitions will say that a fit body is 'sound physically and mentally.' The American College of Sports Medicine (ACSM) is the exercise-science association that sets the standards for exercise physiologists in the United States. The ACSM uses current research to redefine and update its prevention-oriented recommendations for maintaining the body through attention to the components of physical fitness.

The ACSM made the following position statement:

> The Recommended Quantity and Quality of Exercise for Developing and Maintaining Cardiorespiratory and Muscular Fitness, and Flexibility in Healthy Adults.' The ACSM recommends that most adults engage in moderate-intensity cardiorespiratory exercise training for thirty min or more five days/week with vigorous-intensity cardiorespiratory exercise training for twenty minutes or more for three or more days/week, or a combination of moderate-and vigorous-intensity exercise to achieve a total energy expenditure of ≥500–1000 MET·minutes/week. On 2–3 days/week, adults should also perform resistance exercises for each of the major muscle groups, and neuromotor exercise involving balance, agility, and coordination. Crucial to maintaining joint range of movement, completing a series of flexibility exercises for each the major muscle-tendon groups (a total of sixty seconds per exercise) on two or more days/week is recommended. The exercise program should be modified according to an individual's habitual physical activity, physical function, health status, exercise responses, and stated goals. Adults who are unable or unwilling to meet the exercise targets outlined here still can benefit from engaging in amounts of exercise less than recommended. In addition to exercising regularly, there are health benefits in concurrently reducing total time engaged in sedentary pursuits and also by interspersing frequent, short bouts of standing and physical activity between periods of sedentary activity, even in physically active adults.

Based on this position statement and the research backing it, we can see that scientific evidence demonstrating the beneficial effects of exercise is indisputable, and the benefits of exercise far outweigh the risks in most adults. A program of regular exercise that includes cardiorespiratory, resistance, flexibility, and neuromotor exercise training beyond activities of daily living to improve and maintain physical fitness and health is essential for most adults.

Consultations with a medical professional and diagnostic exercise testing for Coronary Heart Disease are useful when clinically indicated but are not recommended for universal screening to enhance the safety of exercise.[3]

Yoga offers much more. In the last two decades, many studies have looked to document the myriad of ways that a consistent and comprehensive yoga practice can bolster fitness. The key words are *consistent* and *comprehensive*. There is a general consensus among most people who understand the physical practice that yoga will improve flexibility, muscular strength and tone, and balance. The surprise is that there is improvement to cardiovascular strength and endurance, lung capacity and concentration. Stamina is included also because of the deep breathing, the practice of Pranayama, meditation, chakra balancing, mudra, mantra and chanting practice, as well as the increased sense of body awareness.

Kathryn Budig explains, "Yoga is the ultimate fitness routine because it builds cardio strength with flow, develops muscular strength with long, strong holds and creates flexibility with almost every pose. It is also completely customizable."[4]

Muscular strength and tone are indicators of the actual strength and endurance of our muscles. We lose muscle tone and mass as we age.

---

3 Garber, Carol Ewing Ph.D., FACSM, (Chair); Blissmer, Bryan Ph.D.; Deschenes, Michael R. PhD, FACSM; Franklin, Barry A. Ph.D., FACSM; Lamonte, Michael J. Ph.D., FACSM; Lee, I-Min M.D., Sc.D., FACSM; Nieman, David C. Ph.D., FACSM; Swain, David P. Ph.D., FACSM; Journal of American College of Sports Medicine, p.51 http://journals.lww.com/acsmmsse/Fulltext/2011/07000/Quantity_and_Quality_of_Exercise_for_Developing.26.aspx; July 2011; Website; April 10, 2016

4 Kathryn Budig, *The Women's Big Book of Yoga* (New York: Rodale Books, 2012), p.25.

Weightlifting exercises are included in yoga, as the weight lifted here is our own body weight. This a great tool for maximizing muscle mass and strength. The load-bearing aspect of weightlifting improves bone density and increases metabolism.

Every pound of muscle burns between 25 to 50 calories per day, so consistency in practicing muscular strengthening exercises is important to maintaining and building overall metabolism. Try the following:

- Chaturangua (Pushup pose)
- Utkatasana (Powerful pose)
- Parivtitta Parsvakonana (Revolved Side Angle pose)
- Adho Mukha Svanasana (Downward Facing Dog pose)

Also include inversions such as Adho Mukha Vrksasana (Handstand) and arm balances like Parsva Bakasana (Side Crane). Studies have shown that weight bearing poses stimulate bone cells to regenerate, thus strengthening bone structure and density.[5]

Yoga clearly improves flexibility both physically and emotionally. Many studies across the world have looked at different aspects of the effects that regular practice have on mobility, regarding both muscular and joint health.

Plants are born tender and pliant; dead, they are brittle and dry. Thus whoever is stiff and inflexible is a disciple of death. Whoever is soft and yielding is a disciple of life. The hard and stiff will be broken. The soft and supple will prevail.
—Lao Tzu

As we age, our bodies are affected by gravity and lack of use; as a result, we grow tighter and shorter. This decreased mobility can lead to chronic pain and injury and can therefore be a downward, repetitive cycle of increased pain and potential injury. Our bodies are intricately designed with many interconnections of function: muscles working synergistically, muscles working to help organ function, and cellular regeneration improving vascular health. A regular yoga asana practice strengthens and elongates muscles, creating space to counter the effects of gravity and promote wellness.

---

5 Dr. Loren Fishman, MD, and Ellen Saltonstall, *Yoga for Osteoporosis*; New York; Norton & Co., 2010

We can use specific poses to isolate muscles that we want to work on, such as using folds to help hamstring and lower back flexibility and twists to help with tension held in spinal muscles. We can address the overall mobility of the body with a comprehensive practice that allows us freedom in all the ways our bodies were meant to move.

The common thread in all the poses is extension of the spine. This is because the action with the alignment of all poses—no matter what the relationship to gravity—is to create space between the vertebrae. This, in turn, allows more space for the discs, more freedom for the nerves that run out from each vertebrae into the body to function optimally, and the smaller muscles that run between the vertebrae to maintain greater muscle fiber length as well as greater strength overall.

Many yogis claim to have "grown" or reclaimed lost height because of their consistent asana practice. Therefore, extension of the spine becomes the fruit of the labor. Twists in yoga create a greater mobility of the spine and rib cage. They bring the blood vessels closer to the disc thus increasing nourishment to the discs, and cleanse the organs with blood perfusion, which happens when coming out of a deep twist. Freedom in the body leads to freedom of mind and spirit, an improvement in self-confidence, and a sense that we are capable of doing what is put before us.

The little space within the heart is as great as the vast universe. The heavens and the earth are there, and the sun and the moon and the stars. Fire and lightning and winds are there, and all that now is and all that is not. —The Upanishads

For decades in the West, the leading cause of death for both men and women has been cardiovascular disease. It is now the leading cause of death worldwide, which is an alarming statistic tied to the effects of the western lifestyle on the global community.

The well-documented risk of heart disease is hard to ignore. Furthermore, so many issues can arise and are grouped into the term, cardiovascular disease (CVD). *Arteriosclerosis*, or hardening of the arteries, includes coronary heart disease, angina, and myocardial infarction. Other issues include *arrhythmias*, which are structural defects such as ventricular septal defects. In addition, there are physical problems that contribute to cardiovascular insufficiency, such as hypertension, strokes, and high cholesterol. Factors that contribute to decreased optimum heart function include elevated triglyceride and homocysteine levels, smoking, obesity, stress, depression, and isolation. Heart health is essential to good health overall and can be accessed with regular exercise, stress management, and proper nutrition.

Optimum heart health—moving blood in and out of the heart, and throughout the body—depends on a strong heart muscle, rhythmic contractions, sound blood vessels, sturdy lungs, and nutrient-rich oxygenated blood. The outcome is nourishment to all body tissues and organs while extracting waste.

Nearly all men and women—no matter their current health conditions—can improve their circulatory systems and function with lifestyle changes to include diet, vitamin supplements, exercise, stress management—particularly yoga and meditation—support groups, and volunteer work. Yoga is helpful in particular because its holistic effect includes attention to the physical, emotional, and spiritual aspects of cardiovascular care.

In 1990, Dean Ornish, MD, and a research team did landmark studies[6] involving diet, yoga, visualization, meditation, group support and other lifestyle changes. Since then, this research has spurred a myriad of other studies. It has become a model for many hospital-based cardiac rehabilitation programs to include yoga and meditation.

Nischala Devi—a published author and yoga teacher who helped design the yoga program for Dr. Dean Ornish's Preventative Medicine Research Institute in Sausalito, CA—explains that healthy heart function not only is a metaphor for balancing how we give and receive, but that it is also unselfish to put ourselves first because the heart feeds

---

6 Dr. Dean Ornish; *"Dr. Dean Ornish's Program for Reversing Heart Disease: the Only System Scientifically Proven to Reverse Heart Disease"*; New York; Random House; 1996

itself first. Furthermore, to live truthfully, to follow your intuition, and to extend yourself to people all lead to heartfelt joy and the feeling of a full and happy heart.

This paramount study led to many more studies, and today many hospital programs incorporate yoga as therapy for cardiovascular patients as a result of the continued discoveries of studies linking cardiovascular benefits with the practice of yoga. At the other end of the scale, professional and Olympic-level teams incorporate a regular practice for their athletes, noting the enhancement to the cardiovascular system, a decrease in sports-related and overuse injuries, and overall well-being—not just the improved muscular and performance benefits.

More recent studies on the effects of yoga for the cardiovascular system have spurred headlines indicating that yoga is as good for your heart as aerobic exercise. Questions of efficacy have raised increased interest to spur more studies. Though yoga's benefits have been long suspected, a study at Harvard University comparing 37 randomized, controlled, clinical trials involving 2,768 people found that the stress reduction and behavior modification benefits that came from a consistent yoga practice positively affected all patients. This was true especially for patients with cardiovascular disease as well as patients with risk factors for metabolic syndrome.[7]

Currently, we understand that yoga is linked to the reduction of several key risk factors of cardiovascular disease including lower body mass index, weight loss, improved cholesterol levels, lower blood pressure, and reduced heart rate. The research does not seem to show much difference in overall cardiovascular benefits when comparing yoga to other forms of aerobic exercise.[8]

---

7 Janice Neumann; *"Yoga may benefit heart health as much as Aerobics"*; http://www.reuters. com/article/2014/12/26/us-health-yoga-cardio-trials-idUSKBN0K40Y520141226? December 2014; April 10, 2016
8 Kay Heagberg; New Study Highlights Yoga's Cardiovascular Benefits; https://yogainternational.com/article/view/new-study-highlights-yogas-cardiovascular-benefits; February 2015; Website; April 10, 2016

If yoga and heart health are of interest to you, we encourage you to do your own further research in this area. Interestingly, studies done on this topic have not used the same styles of yoga asana practice, so we cannot link the effects to a certain way of practicing yoga. Also consistent with studies analyzing benefits of yoga is the finding that yoga provides emotional and spiritual benefits including stress reduction, self-recognition, and an overall sense of well-being and connectedness/support.

Yoga has a sly, clever way of short circuiting the mental patterns that cause anxiety.
—Baxter Bell

In the scientific arena, it is accepted that there is a need for aerobic exercise to challenge and strengthen the heart muscle, to help the supporting blood vessels be more resilient, to enhance the overall health of the body due to efficient cardiovascular function, and for the body to be prepared for stress physically. Consistent yoga practice seems to bring a more comprehensive healing effect of the heart. This is because yoga opens the heart chakra that leads to the opening of the body, mind, and spirit.

Yoga and Brain Chemistry

For centuries, yogis have known that their practice does wonders for the mind. Whether one or all three of the following are practiced—asana (physical postures), pranayama (breath work), and meditation—there is increased cognitive ability, mental stability, clarity, and ease of mental and emotional stress—both during and after practice.

Given the steady rise in the number of people practicing yoga—from 13 million in 2007 to more than 20 million today—researchers have begun to focus their attention on how yoga actually changes the brain. Studies show that yoga increases relaxation in the brain, improves areas of the brain that help us manage pain, and protect us against age-related decline.[9]

---

9 Heagberg, Kat; *This is Your Brain on Yoga; https://yogainternational.com/article/view/this-is-your-brain-on-yoga*; January 2014; Website; April 20, 2016

Modern medicine—including the use of brain imaging technologies—is validating what yogis have been experiencing for centuries: truly, yogic practices can change your brain. As we consider modern advances in neuroscience related to the brain's anatomy and function, we can begin to understand the deeper meaning of "mind-body."

Bo Forbes—a clinical psychologist and integrative yoga therapist—explains, "the cerebrum, the largest part of your brain, is considered the "seat of conscious functioning."" Physically, the right hemisphere controls the left side of the body, and the left hemisphere controls the right. Regarding the five sheaths of the body, on the level of the subtle body, *ida nadi* (the lunar energy channel) is connected to the right half of the brain, and *pingala nadi* (the solar energy channel) is connected to the left side of the brain. Bo Forbes's work and interest in *neuroplasticity* (the ability to change our emotional and mental habits) take into account that the mind-body network includes the following systems, pathways, and so on:

- Nervous system
- Emotional body (limbic system)
- Immune system
- Enteric nervous system (the belly brain)
- Pain regulation pathways
- Deep visceral body (the primal and nonverbal body—the seat of wisdom, intuition, and creativity)

In her work, Bo Forbes also explains, "The anterior part of the frontal lobe, the prefrontal cortex, is the most evolved part of the brain and is responsible for positive capacities like concentration, happiness, creativity, and rational thinking. Studies using EEG have shown that meditation strengthens communication between the prefrontal cortex and other areas of the brain."[10]

---

10 See footnote 9

The practice of mindfulness meditation is growing with great momentum as the Western world has realized the usefulness of slowing the pace of life intentionally. Many studies are looking to understand the myriad of positive effects of mindfulness meditation that have come to include reducing cognitive stress, decreasing stress arousal and depression, shifting perspective, providing clarity, increasing positive states of mind, and promoting hormonal changes that enhance physical-body mechanics. Furthermore, recent scientific studies are documenting the effects of mindfulness meditation on potential longevity by studying telomere length, the protective caps at the end of chromosomes.[11]

The concept of neuroplasticity is accepted readily in the yoga therapy community where there is recognition of the capacity to work against *samskaras*, or negative habits. We do not want to "deepen the grooves" of the old samskaras. We can repeat healthier habits in what we do (asana and pranayama practice, tasks of daily living, dietary choices, and so on), what we say (stopping to think before reacting, using more positive words, how we nurture our relationships and so on), and what we think (using sound healing, mantras, visualization, and aromatherapy) to affect mood, and mindfulness practices. We can begin to replace the old, default habits with new patterns that contribute to our well-being. In the area of neuroscience, it is recognized that the more an activity and/or a behavior is repeated, the more neural connections are forged; neural links are then strengthened.

The seven chakras of the body are associated with many different body parts, organ systems, colors, and emotions that help improve physical, emotional and spiritual health. Your asana practice helps keep open the channels and energy associated with each chakra thus enabling their healthy function. Much study, especially self-study, is

---

11 Eppel, Elisa; Daubenmier, Jennifer; Moskowitz, Judith; Folkman, Susan; Blackbourn, Elizabeth; *Can Meditation Slow Rate of Cellular Aging; Cognitve Stress, Mindfulness, and Telomeres; Annals of the NY Academy of Sciences;* onlinelibrary.wiley.com/doi/10.1111/j.1749-6632.2009.04414.x/abstract; August, 2009; April 10, 2016

spent focusing on the chakra system. The sixth chakra—Ajna chakra (known as the third eye)—is located in the center of the forehead. It is associated with the pituitary gland and is considered the "command center" of the mind despite its rather small size. Physiologically, the pituitary gland reins as the endocrine system's master gland because it produces and releases hormones to control growth, metabolism, and overall body function.

The brain's messengers—*neurotransmitters*—relay information between brain and nerve cells. Neurological disorders are often the result of neurotransmitter issues. Low levels of the neurotransmitter, GABA, are associated with depression and anxiety. Many studies are underway to document the physiological and biomechanical benefits of yoga. Studies show a correlation between consistent asana practice and increased GABA levels.[12]

The *brain stem* connects the brain and the spinal cord, aids in digestion, heart rate, and diaphragmatic breathing. Neurons from the brain stem send a nerve impulse to the diaphragm, which causes it to contract, thereby initiating inhalation. Though this is an involuntary action of the body, respiration can also be a voluntary action. An average person takes about 12 breaths per minute if he or she does not "watch the breath." Once we bring our attention to our breathing, we begin to take slower, fuller breaths automatically. This happens in many breathing exercises in pranayama and meditation. Physiologically, the advantages include increased lung capacity as well as stronger and more flexible muscles of respiration (intercostal muscles, diaphragm, and abdominal wall).

Once we create a pattern of a longer exhalation compared to the inhalation, we turn off our body's "fight or flight" mechanism, which the sympathetic nervous system places in overdrive. This allows the parasympathetic nervous system to override the sympathetic nervous

---

12 Heagberg, Kat; *This is Your Brain on Yoga; https://yogainternational.com/article/view/this-is-your-brain-on-yoga*; January 2014; Website; April 20, 2016

system with the following advantages: lowered heart rate and blood pressure, slower muscle-fiber twitch, decreased respiration, reduced perspiration, and a general lowered sense of anxiety.

The *frontal lobe* of the brain handles higher cognitive functions—planning, discriminating, abstract thinking, personality, and behavior. In Ayurvedic practices, breathing practices rejuvenate and purify this area of the brain.

The *cerebellum* controls balance, muscle coordination, reflexes, and movement. It is necessary for execution of all asana practice and also improves with consistent asana practice.

The *limbic system* consists of the hippocampus, amygdala, thalamus, and hypothalamus, which integrate memory and emotion into the physical body. The practice of meditation has been shown in many studies to reduce gray matter in the amygdala (linked to fear and anxiety). Meditation has also been shown to increase gray matter in the hippocampus, which plays a vital role in memory formation.

Aromatherapy has great effects on the limbic system—especially when certain scents are tied to memory, even when we are not aware of the connection of the memory and the aroma. We can affect mood by using essential oils that are known to be calming, invigorating, or energizing. For example, mint oils are typically rich in ketones and are thus energizing. Citrus oils contain high levels of monoterpenes and are uplifting. Spices with aldehydes and phenols are invigorating. Florals have high alcohol content and are known for their calming and soothing properties. Typically, trees, herbs, and grass oils are rich in esters and oxides, making them renewing and relaxing.

It's important to recognize that in spite of these generalized benefits, each person will respond differently to individual essential oils or blends because of physiological variants. So, as we use essential oils, we can experiment with various ones to see how we will respond *personally.* Our memories, too, will help direct which oils will work more effectively for each person. Our dosha/constitution and our past experiences tied to memory will couple with certain choices for use of effective aromatherapy.

The primary visual processing center of the brain—the *occipital lobe*—helps us visually in yoga class. Using our focusing skills helps to refine balance and vice versa. Headstand is said to improve visual acuity. The *temporal lobe* is responsible for auditory perception such as hearing the cues of your yoga teacher. Shoulder stand helps sharpen hearing acuity and incidentally, it also helps enhance thyroid function.

The *parietal lobe* governs limb movement, speech, and sensory feedback. Many studies in this area hope to encourage the practice of yoga in clinical settings to help clients manage pain. The combination of an asana practice to work off negative energy/stress using breathing techniques and especially the learned cognitive practices in yoga (feeling the pain and detaching from the emotion behind it) have proven helpful in teaching clients to tolerate their pain with ease. One study even discovered that yogis—compared to a control group—could tolerate their pain twice as long.[13]

A consistent yoga practice that includes asana, pranayama, and meditation provides many comprehensive benefits to our brain and nervous system. A growing body of research in the area of yoga in the West has shown us that it does in fact affect brain function. This has sparked interest and action in the areas of science and medicine so that more recent and future studies are looking more specifically to "how" it works.

Summary
The effects of a yoga practice invoke relaxation by stimulating the parasympathetic nervous system, improving regions of the brain that

13 Edwards, Alan; *Insular cortex mediates increased pain tolerance in yoga practitioners*; US National Library of Medicine National Institutes of Health; http://www.ncbi.nlm.nih.gov/pubmed/23696275; May, 2013; April 10, 2016

manage pain, protecting against age-related decline such as fluid intelligence and cognitive flexibility, and improving mindfulness. The benefits of yoga are not just for healthy people, but also for clinical populations. Those with physical limitations, emotional issues such as depression and anxiety, and cognitive impairments such as dementia are included. This general fine-tuning of the body, mind, and spirit can be enhanced further by complimenting the yoga practice with pure and potent essential oils.

Whenever you consider beginning a new facet or activity to support the healthy function of your body, it is wise to consult with your licensed health-care provider to ensure that these practices and activities are best for you and your specific situation.

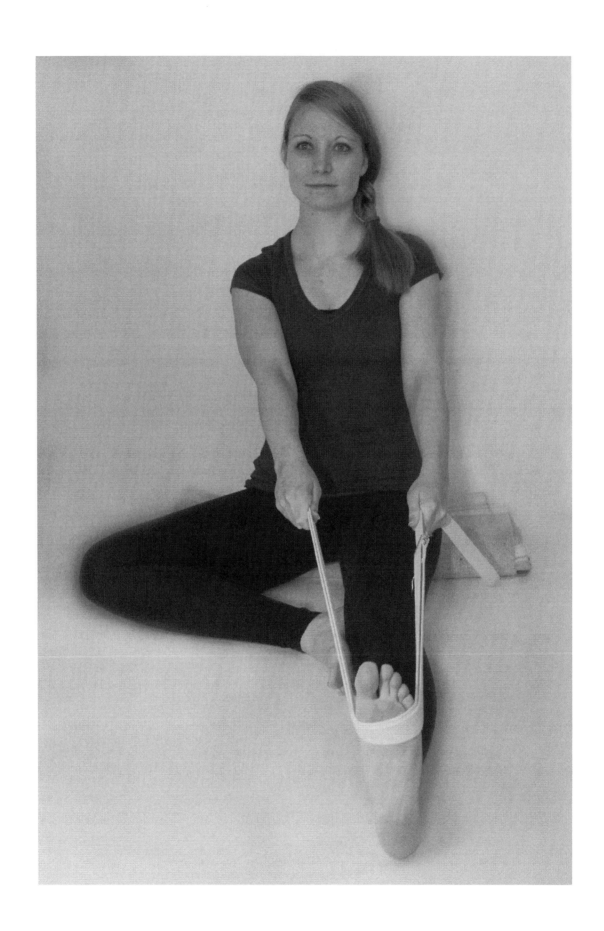

SECTION 6: YOGA TIPS

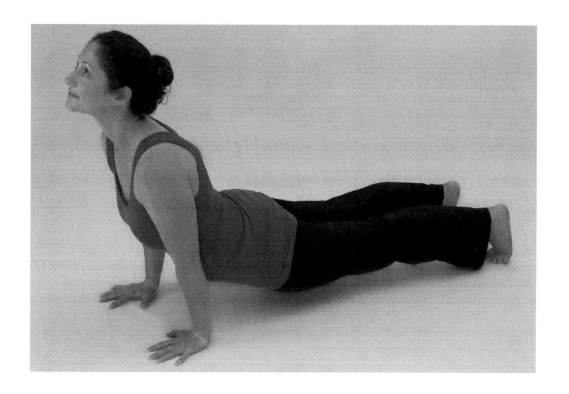

This yoga should be practiced with firm determination and perseverance, without any mental reservation or doubts. — Bhagavad Gita

Tip #1

Generally, yoga practice is done in bare feet. The standing poses provide an improved agility of the feet and ankles, and there are many correlations to improved mobility of the spine and rib cage as a result. Humility, respect, and regard to cleanliness are the reasons one removes their shoes at the door of the yoga practice room for a group practice. Standing poses are also very grounding and build resilience of core strength and balance, so bare-feet practice will enhance those outcomes.

Tip #2

A greeting with hands in prayer position, held at the heart chakra, is also very traditional, both at the beginning and at the end of the practice. The heart is the "seat of our intuition," as explained by B. K. S. Iyengar. Hands joined together at the heart is called "Anjali Mudra" or "Namaskarasana." This gesture symbolizes respect and union. "Namaste" is the greeting used to end the practice but can be used at the beginning of the practice as well. This single word has great meaning and has been translated in many ways, but its essence is a sign of respect to honor the practice of yoga—everyone practicing together, the teacher and the teacher's lineage.

My first teacher used the following translation of the word *Namaste*: "The honor in me respects the honor in you, as we have come to work together in harmony." This paints a much bigger picture and puts great responsibility in the hands of all practicing together to honor one another, to be stewards of the practice, while working together with good intentions.

Tip #3

Another traditional part of yoga is to chant, both at the beginning and at the end of the practice. For some in the West, it is hard to grasp this idea as necessary, especially if traditional chants are used, when most people might not know the meaning of the Sanskrit words in the chant.

Most traditional teachers use certain chants that come from the practice of their yoga lineage. This is another way to honor their teachers. The word, *OM (or OHM)*, represents the sound of the universe and the practice of chanting OM three times at the beginning and at the end of class incorporates many other ideas. As it is the sound of the universe, it connects us to our world and thus is very grounding. It binds together the people in the room practicing and seals the practice at

Kindness and awareness work together. Through awareness we understand the underlying beauty of everything and every being.
—Amit Ray

Chanting is a way of getting in touch with yourself. It's an opening of the heart and letting go of the mind and thoughts. It deepens the channel of grace, and it's a way of being present in the moment.
—Krishna Das

the end. It opens the lungs and prepares the rib cage, lungs, and diaphragm for asana practice.

As three deep breaths are necessary to chant these three OMs, deep breathing quiets the mind and allows the students to focus on the present moment and on the practice before them. It allows quieting of mind chatter and a break from this habit that builds our stress. If it seems odd at first, just sit quietly and enjoy the vibrational energy that comes from a group chant.

Vibrational energy is also very healing on a physical, emotional, and spiritual level. One option is to hold your hand on your heart to feel the vibration of the chant. Some groups—especially church yoga classes— opt to chant, *AHMEN*, or *SHALOM*, which has the same root word and provides all of the same benefits.

On another note, it is considered among the first sounds that a baby can make. Babies open their mouths and say, "AAHHH," which is much like, "OOOOHHH." To close the mouth and finish sound, there is a sound, "MMMM." Usually, the first word that a baby says is, "MAMA." These initial sounds begin language development and are universal.

In addition to OM, mantras are chanted. *Mantras* are words or phrases that are repeated with the ideal that the mindset will be affected through the repeated listening of the sound. "Man" refers to the mind and "tra" means wave. The meaning of the word(s) chanted is projected to the mind.

The vibrational energy of the chant is very healing, and sound vibration affects body, mind, and spirit. The meridian points on the roof of the mouth can direct this vibrational energy to change the chemistry of the brain and can be very energizing or soothing. The meaning of different mantras can direct a distinct energetic state but ultimately, all mantras lead us to a deeper connection with ourselves. They pave the way to transcending the typical mind chatter, becoming attuned to our inherent gifts, and connecting to our Higher Power. This is another way yogis can feel that their yoga practice deepens their faith practice.

Tip #4

Yoga is not a religious practice, but rather a spiritual practice. Remember, *yoga* means to yoke and is a union of body, mind, and spirit. Because it originated in India, it is often associated with the Hindu religion, including the fact that several poses are named for Hindu deities. However, yoga was originally introduced in the *Vedas*, which came long before the Hindu religion. There are usually wonderful stories that provide great life lessons, great positive energy, and can contribute to an energetic opening of the chakras for that particular pose. There may be representations of Hindu deities in many yoga studios, and usually they are very ornamental.

Learning some of the stories lends itself to the practice in general. For example, Ganesha is "the destroyer of obstacles." Thinking of Ganesha may help you get through a challenging pose. Warrior poses are meant to provide a sense of readiness and are generally used ahead of more challenging poses. Twists were named for sages. The wisdom that comes from inward reflection accessed in a twist can lead to a significant release or "squeezing out" of unnecessary ideas and tension by going into a twist. There is also an analogy in coming out of a twist: there is newfound freedom as the body unwinds—in many aspects—in body, mind, and spirit.

Tip #5

All action in yoga is light and there is a balance of "opposing" actions in every pose. One should never force movement, breath, or move in a way that goes against intuition. On the other hand, keeping an open mind to new movements and poses may yield a pleasant surprise: you are stronger than you think! You will build not just body awareness, but also an ability to trust your body as you build strength and resilience. Therefore, a consistent yoga practice can be rather empowering.

If I'm losing balance in a pose, I stretch higher and God reaches down to steady me. It works every time, and not just in yoga.
—Terri Guillemets

Don't seek, don't search, don't ask, don't knock, don't demand ~ relax. If you relax, it comes. If you relax, it is there. If you relax, you start vibrating with it.
—Osho

Namaste: *I honor the Place in You in which the entire universe dwells. I honor the Place in You which is of love, of truth, of light and of Peace. When You are in that Place in You and I am in that Place in me, we are one.*

Tip #6

The meaning of "Namaste" is comprehensive and universal. Traditionally, one brings together the hands, in a prayer position, at the heart chakra, with the head bowed. It can also be initiated by bringing together the hands at the third eye—the Ajna chakra—which signifies clear vision, and then moving the hands down, in front of the heart.

Aadil Palkhivala, founder of Purna Yoga and a world-renowned teacher, explains that it is a gesture of respect, both toward the self and the teacher or group. It represents recognition of the divine spark that resides in the heart chakra. Namaste is also an acknowledgment of the soul of one to the soul of another.

Namaste is an ultimate form of respect of two or more people coming together energetically, free from the bonds of ego, thus allowing a great purpose to form and bloom from the collective time and work together. As mentioned earlier, typically, it is used both at the beginning and at the end of a group practice. More often, it is used just at the end to seal the practice.

The teacher will initiate the gesture, to show respect to his/her students and to recognize the lineage of their practice. The student(s) return the gesture. In the East, the gesture needs no spoken word. In the West, we have adopted both doing and saying, "Namaste." *Nama* means bow, *as* means I, and *te* means you. Literally then, *Namaste* means, "I bow to you."

Essential oils have been around since the beginning of time, and—like yoga—have been used to support physical, emotional, and mental wellness for centuries.

Study nature, love nature, stay close to nature. It will never fail you.
—Frank Lloyd Wright

All essential oils are not sourced, extracted, and processed to be an equal grade. The next section gives further clarity about essential oils. It discusses what a yoga studio might look for to ensure that the essential oils used would benefit their yogis rather than impact the yoga experience and result negatively. (For more information about this particular topic, see the "Sourcing, Extracting, and Harvesting Procedures" section on page 71.)

PART 2: ESSENTIAL OILS

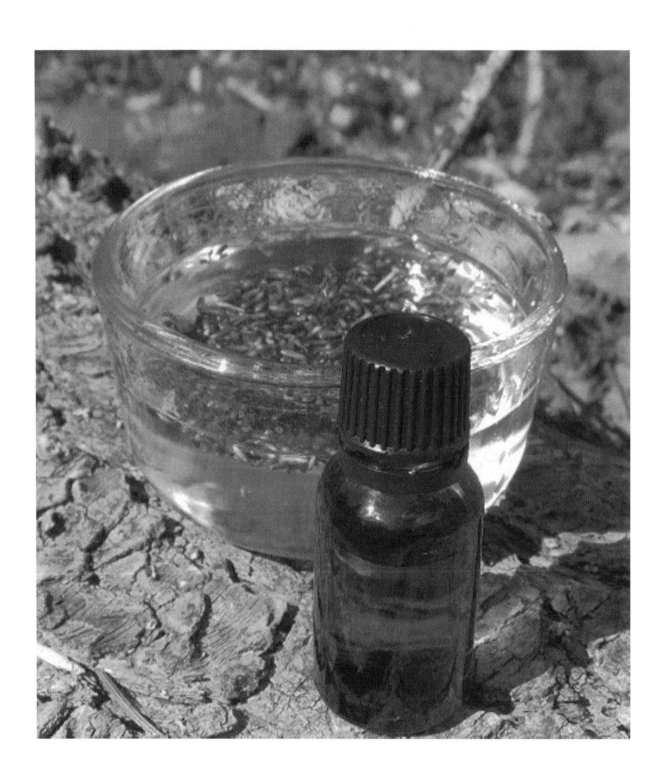

SECTION 7: ESSENTIAL OILS— WHAT THEY ARE AND HOW THEY BENEFIT US

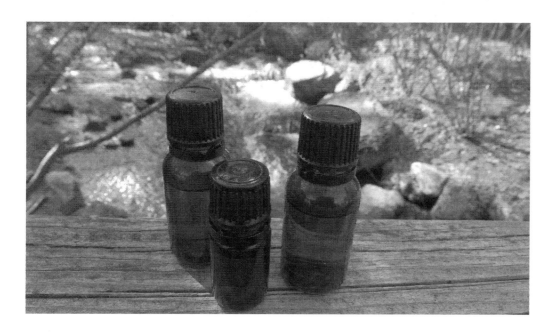

Those who find beauty in all of nature will find themselves at one with the secrets of life itself. —L. W. Gilbert

What are essential oils?

Essential oils are aromatic, volatile compounds found in plants. In this case, *volatile* means that essential oils evaporate easily. Essential oils are different than fixed oils. An example of a fixed oil is olive oil, which is much heavier, contains fatty acids, and feels oily to the touch. When you walk past a bed of roses and smell the beautiful scent in the air, it is rose essential oil that you are smelling. "The term 'essential oil' is a contraction of the original 'quintessential oil.' This stems from the Aristotelian idea that matter is composed of four elements, namely, fire, air, earth, and water. The fifth element, or quintessence, was then considered to be spirit or life force. Distillation and evaporation were thought to be processes of removing the spirit from the plant and this is also reflected in our language since the term 'spirits' is used to describe distilled alcoholic beverages such as brandy, whiskey, and eau de vie. The last of these again shows reference to the concept of removing the life force from the plant. Nowadays, of course, we know that, far from being spirit, essential oils are physical in nature and composed of complex mixtures of chemicals."[14]

Each essential oil is comprised of aromatic compounds that have certain characteristics. These compounds help the plant to thrive in its environment in a number of ways. First of all, they can help protect the plant from environmental threats. They can also attract pollinators—a critical element in the survival of plant species.

Conversely, the aromatic compounds can also repel certain animals and insects. Due to the tiny molecular size of these compounds, we can benefit greatly from 100-percent *pure* essential oils (which means they are carbon based, like us). This is why they are able to penetrate cells and tissues very quickly and support our bodies on a cellular level.

Essential oils are located in specific sacs or ducts on the plant, and they are highly concentrated. Depending on the plant, they can be found in the roots, leaves, flowers, seeds, or bark of the plant. The amount of essential oil that can be extracted from a plant varies greatly. For example, it takes around four thousand pounds of roses to make one pound of rose oil (about thirty roses to make a single drop). It takes about 150 pounds of lavender to produce one pound of lavender oil. Pure essential oils are compatible for use by humans and many animals. As

---

14 Charles Sell, "The Chemistry of Essential Oils," *Handbook of Essential Oils: Science, Technology, and Applications* (Boca Raton: CRC Press, 2010), 121–150.

nature's creation, they are perfectly formed and can benefit us with general and targeted supplemental support for healthy physical and emotional function.

How Do Essential Oils Benefit Us?

Physical Wellness:

Essential oils are a natural way to enhance our health and wellness. The compounds that make up essential oils are known for providing a variety of benefits that support the healthy structure and function of body parts and systems. For example, *esters* are typically soothing and calming. *Monoterpenes* can be uplifting and energizing. *Ketones* have properties that are typically supportive of a healthy integumentary system. As mentioned earlier, essential oils are comprised of these, and/or many other possible compounds in a variety of combinations. Not only do the combinations vary, but the amount of each compound in an essential oil also varies. The overall benefit of the essential oil is derived from how these compounds work together in a synergistic way.

Vitality and beauty are gifts of Nature for those who live according to its laws.
—Leonardo Da Vinci

Body Systems Support:

Because essential oils support the healthy functions of the body, it is helpful to have a working knowledge of the body systems and what they do for us. See the following body system summary:

Take care of your body. It's the only place you have to live.
—Jim Rohn

- Respiratory System
    - Helps supply the blood with oxygen (keeps our cells alive and healthy)
    - Helps release carbon dioxide from the body
- Digestive System
    - Helps us break down and utilize nutrients we receive from our food
- Cardiovascular/Circulatory System
    - Lungs, heart, and the rest of the system work together consistently to pump life-giving blood through our body

- Endocrine System
  - A complex system of glands (separate but interrelated) that each secrete different hormones that control and coordinate body functions. These hormones (chemical substances) affect and regulate mood, sleep, metabolism, growth, reproduction, and sexual function. An example of a hormone that affects the body is *insulin*, which controls blood sugar levels.
  - Impacts almost every cell and organ in the body directly
  - Some of the major glands in this system are:
    - Adrenal glands (secrete adrenaline, which in turn has a direct effect on heart rate and blood pressure)
    - Thyroid (regulates how the body burns fuel)
    - Parathyroids (regulate calcium in the blood)
    - Pineal gland (secretes *melatonin*, which helps regulate sleep)
    - Hypothalamus (connects the endocrine system with the nervous system)
    - Pituitary gland (makes hormones that control the other endocrine glands; most important gland in the endocrine system)
    - Reproductive gland (primary source of sex hormones)
- Excretory System
  - Causes the body to locate and remove dangerous poisons, waste materials, and toxins from the body. Liquid waste is processed through the kidneys. Gas waste is carried to the lungs and exhaled from the body. Dead cells and sweat are released through the skin (part of the integumentary system).
- Integumentary System
  - Works together with the excretory system to remove surface-level waste. It also protects inner organs and systems. Skin, hair, toenails, and fingernails comprise this system.
- Urinary System

- ○ Includes ureters, kidneys, urethra, bladder, and sphincter muscles that work together to create, carry and store urine
- Lymphatic & Immune System
  - ○ Helps create immune cells
  - ○ Helps absorb and move fat to the circulatory system
  - ○ Helps protect the body from infection, microorganisms/germs, and disease
- Limbic and Nervous System
  - ○ Forms and regulates emotions and holds our memories (limbic system). The autonomic nervous system involves sympathetic and parasympathetic responses (fight or flight response). While emotions are regulated by the entire nervous system, the limbic system and autonomic nervous system are particularly important.
  - ○ Central Nervous System: coordinated by the brain. It receives information from various parts of the body and interprets that information to help the body function (think, remember, react, and so on).
  Peripheral Nervous System (PNS): carries the information back to our brain; we send messages when we move our muscles and joints. Part of the PNS is the autonomic nervous system, which manages functions such as digestion.

Our bodies are designed to be healthy when they receive proper care and nutrition. It is easy to see how the body systems are interconnected. It is exciting to learn about the science of essential oils and how the chemical compounds within essential oils can work with us to supplement our efforts in supporting the healthy functioning of our bodies.

Because essential oils vary in their benefits and the support they provide to the body, we highly recommend that you do your own research from reputable sources to find out more about how to use specific essential oils to support your wellness goals. Some common uses for healthy-body system support by essential oils include the following:

Nature spontaneously keeps us well. Do not resist her!
—Henry David Thoreau

Respiratory System

- Help maintain feelings of clear breathing
- Help maintain respiratory health

Digestive System

- May help ease occasional indigestion
- May help support healthy digestion
- May help reduce feelings of bloating and gas
- Soothe occasional stomach discomfort
- Support healthy metabolic function
- Cleanse the body naturally and aid in healthy digestion
- Help manage hunger cravings
- Help calm the stomach

Cardiovascular/ Circulatory System

- Maintain healthy circulation
- May promote healthy cardiovascular system function
- Support cardiovascular health

Endocrine System

- Help balance mood throughout the month

Excretory System

- (See Digestive System and Integumentary System)

Integumentary System

- Act as a cooling agent for the skin
- Help reduce the appearance of blemishes
- May have purifying and/or clarifying benefits for skin

- Promote healthy hair and scalp
- May have a calming, soothing effect on skin
- Natural skin toner
- Beneficial for oily skin conditions
- May help improve the appearance of oily skin
- May help rejuvenate skin
- Help keep skin clean, clear, and hydrated
- Help sustain smoother, more radiant skin
- Nourish and protect skin and scalp
- May help purify and tone skin
- Help balance moisture levels in the skin
- May reduce appearance of scars and blemishes

Urinary System

- Support healthy kidney and urinary tract function

Lymphatic and Immune System

- Help minimize the effects of seasonal threats
- May help support healthy immune system function
- May protect against environmental and seasonal threats
- Help support the body's natural antioxidant defenses

Limbic and Nervous System

- May help with feelings of mental clarity
- May assist with a sense of openness and a clear head

This is powerful! As we become more familiar with the properties and benefits of various constituents found in essential oils, we can more effectively use essential oils as a supplemental natural support to our wellness goals.

Keep in mind that essential oils are extremely concentrated. This means that, in most situations, only 1–2 drops can help provide the targeted support you are seeking. This means that they are incredibly inexpensive. The bottom line is that using all-natural essential oils is safe, inexpensive, *and* effective. They have been used for centuries to support individuals all over the globe, and now it's our turn to enjoy their benefits.

Focus and Concentration

That's been one of my mantras—focus and simplicity. Simple can be harder than complex: You have to work hard to get your thinking clean to make it simple. But it's worth it in the end because once you get there, you can move mountains.
—Steve Jobs

When we use essential oils aromatically, the first system to come into contact with the essential oils is our *olfactory* system (we smell them). Our nasal cavities have olfactory nerves that are connected to the olfactory bulb located in the back of the nose. The olfactory bulb is able to bypass the conscious brain and send messages directly to the limbic system.

Smelling a fragrance is not only a fast way to get a message to the brain, it is also one of the most powerful. We retain powerful memories associated with the sense of smell. Think back to certain aromas from your childhood—did you ever come home from school when bread or chocolate chip cookies were baking in the oven? Do you associate a cinnamon/citrus smell, commonly used in Wassail during December holidays, with a cozy feeling of home?

The limbic system is the part of the brain that stores memories, emotions, and is also involved in learning and memory. It influences the endocrine system and autonomic nervous system in the body. This is a powerful player in our body chemistry as well as emotional and physiological well-being.

Think of the power of using all-natural essential oils to support healthy cognitive functions including focus, concentration, energy level and/or ability to stay on task. Reference the Body System and Essential Oil list in the preceding section for a more comprehensive overview of how essential oils can support the healthy functioning of our limbic and nervous systems.

Emotional Wellness

We have talked a lot about physical benefits of using essential oils. Another major benefit comes in the form of emotional support. Some essential oils have properties that help calm and soothe emotions, uplift and invigorate emotions, and help support overall feelings of balance and well-being.

When it comes to emotional wellness, we can add the following essential oil benefits to our Body System and Essential Oil list mentioned earlier:

Inhale, and God approaches you. Hold the inhalation, and God remains with you. Exhale, and you approach God. Hold the exhalation, and surrender to God.
—Krishnamacharya

Limbic and Nervous System

- May help relax the mind and body
- Help evoke feelings of tranquility and balance
- Help soothe anxious feelings
- May promote feelings of relaxation
- May help balance mood
- May help soothe occasional feelings of irritability
- Often used in meditation for grounding and uplifting properties
- May help promote a positive outlook

Summary

In other words, essential oils simply support the healthy emotional function of our limbic and nervous systems. Imagine adding a layer of natural support to all your daily activities by simply putting a drop of essential oil in your hands, rubbing them together, and cupping your nose to inhale the beautiful aroma—or by using a diffuser in your home or yoga studio. (A *diffuser* is a machine that vibrates many times per second in order to break down and distribute essential oils into the air, so they can benefit everyone in the immediate environment.) Is there anything on the list above from which you wouldn't want to benefit?

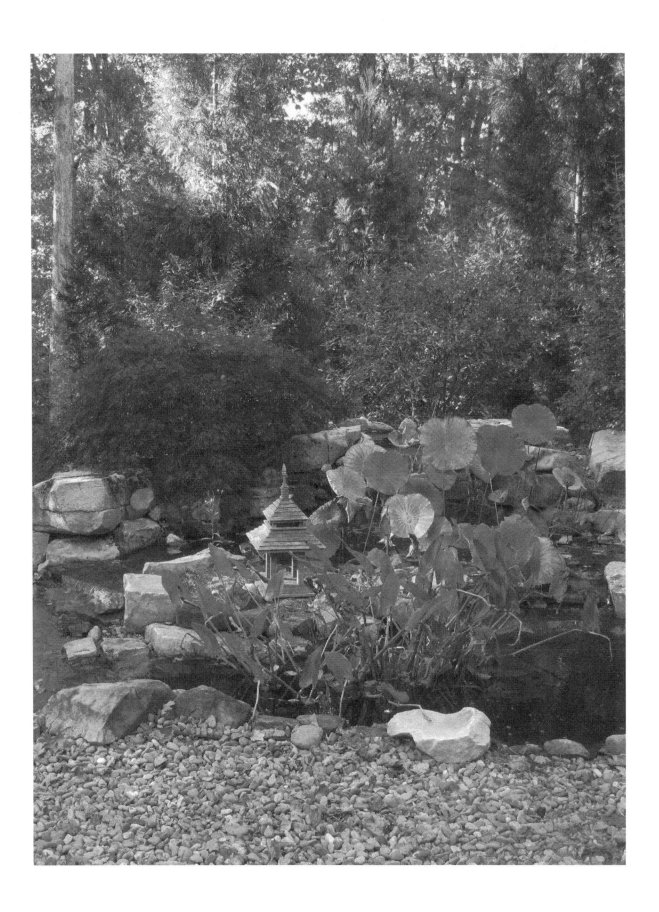

SECTION 8: ESSENTIAL OILS— SOURCING, HARVESTING AND EXTRACTION PROCEDURES

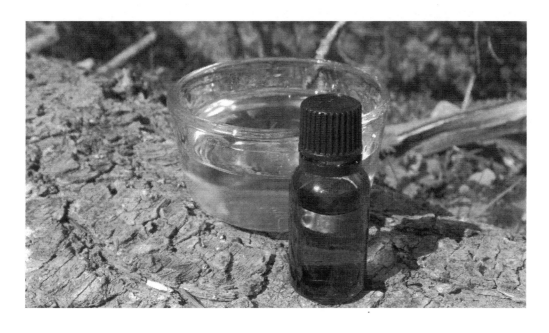

Vitality and beauty are gifts of Nature for those who live according to its laws. —Leonardo Da Vinci

It is important to recognize that not all essential oils are equal in purity or potency. What, exactly, do purity and potency mean? How do they affect the end results of essential oils?

Purity

Purity refers to the percentage of pure, aromatic compounds that comprise an essential oil. This can be difficult to measure because there are no current regulatory standards for "100 percent pure therapeutic grade

Rare is the union of beauty and purity. —Juzenal

essential oil." Needless to say, this can cause great confusion for consumers who desire to use a pure essential oil.

There are three main ways that "purity" of an essential oil can be adulterated:

First, less-expensive synthetic fragrances may be used to dilute, supplement, or replace natural fragrances. Synthetic fragrances are often much more consistent than natural fragrances because the exact fragrance can be duplicated time and time again.

Second, chemicals or pesticides that plants are exposed to may make their way into the essential oil to the detriment of the end-user.

Third, "fillers" may be added. This can include diluting the essential oil in a base of oil (such as fractionated coconut oil, grapeseed oil, or almond oil). Diluting an oil doesn't diminish purity in and of itself, and may actually have benefits for topical use. The end-user would simply want that information for considerations such as shelf life. For example, it would be useful to know whether the base oil will go rancid. Also, if the end-user would like to use that bottle of oil in the future, it would be helpful to know if he or she should further dilute the oil, or whether it is diluted to maximum effectiveness already.

Remember that originally, essential oils are created in "nature's laboratory" by plants themselves. When a *whole* essential oil is created by the plant, we have the assurance that every compound comprising the oil creates a *perfect balance*. When we add to that or take away from it either unintentionally or for our own purposes, the end result can create confusion in our body and reduce the effectiveness of the oil.

Nature does not hurry, yet everything is accomplished.
—Lao Tzu

Potency

Potency refers to the strength of the oil and also the interdependent percentages of chemical compounds that comprise the oil. The existence and percentages of chemical compounds create an overall synergistic effect that determines the strength or potency of any given essential oil.

Note: It is impossible to have a potent oil unless is it pure.

Some of the factors that impact the potency and benefits of an essential oil include the following:

- **Sourcing/geographical location**: The geographical location where plants are sourced has a huge effect on the ultimate chemical footprint of each essential oil. Typically, plants that are grown in their indigenous habitat have a higher potency than their counterparts.[15]
- **Time of harvest—year**: Time of harvest greatly affects the overall composition of an essential oil.[16]
- **Time of harvest—day**: The time of day that some plants are harvested, as well as the drying time of the plant, can also make a difference in the overall chemical composition of the oil.
- **Method of extraction**: There are several methods for extracting essential oils, and some are better than others for different plants. Some of the more common methods are steam distillation and cold-press. Choosing the appropriate extraction method for each plant can be a crucial element in obtaining a truly superior essential oil.
- **Quality of extraction**: Extracting essential oils is an art form based in science, and it requires experts to do it correctly. It is important to perform the extraction at the right temperature so that precious chemical properties of the essential oils stay intact.

---

15 Selvam, Kandasamy. "Antioxidant Potential and Secondary Metabolites in Ocimum Sanctum L. at Various Habitats." *Www.academicjournals.com.* Journal of Medicinal Plants Research, 25 Mar. 2013. Web. 26 Apr. 2016. <http://www.academicjournals.org/journal/JMPR/article-full-text-pdf/C6180C721710>.

16 Turek, Claudia. "Stability of Essential Oils: A Review."*Http://onlinelibrary.wiley.com/.* Comprehensive Reviews in Food Science and Food Safety, 3 Jan. 2013. Web. 26 Apr. 2016. <http://onlinelibrary.wiley.com/doi/10.1111/1541-4337.12006/full>.

What is a consumer to do? How do we know which essential oils are truly pure? If they are pure, how do we know their potency? How can we find an essential oil of superior quality?

The answers lie in testing. The only way to know what you have is to test it, and even testing procedures can differ greatly depending on the experience of the technician and the quality of the testing equipment.

Besides testing, we can also use best consumer practices to gain clues to the safety of the oil. For example, if you go to a health food store and see peppermint oil for sale, check the label! We know peppermint is edible. So, if the oil is pure and has been tested to alleviate all doubt, the bottle label should read accordingly. But if it says, "Not for internal use," there may be cause to question the sourcing, harvesting, extraction, or testing procedures used for that particular peppermint oil.

Authors' Suggestions to Essential Oil Consumers

Change is not something that we should fear. Rather, it is something that we should welcome. For without change, nothing in this world would ever grow or blossom, and no one in this world would ever move forward to become the person they're meant to be.
—Author unknown

With the vast number of companies and holistic healers who work with either middlemen, direct growers, or who grow their own plants to extract essential oils, it can be a confusing and difficult process to select essential oils that are truly pure and potent. In addition, currently, there are no regulatory organizations to help consumers determine which essential oils have the characteristics they seek. Indeed, this would be a daunting task for any governing body because a company is only as trustworthy as its individual batches, which can change drastically due to a number of factors.

To assist you in your essential oil selection process, we have compiled a list of considerations:

- Does the essential oil company you are considering guarantee all of its oils to be pure and potent, 100 percent natural, and without synthetics, chemicals, pesticides or fillers?

- Does your company guarantee that its pure essential oils have a consistent chemical composition from batch to batch?
- Are the essential oils you are considering sourced from various geographical locations around the world where the respective plants are grown indigenously? (This gets you a step closer to finding a chemical footprint ideal to support the healthy function of body systems and structures.)
- Is your company able to identify a consistent "chemical footprint" of each essential oil based on comparison with a vast essential oil database to ensure not only consistency, but also potency for targeted body-system wellness support?
- Are your essential oils harvested at the right time of year and the right time of day to ensure maximum potency and efficacy?
- Does the essential oil company you are considering support the families of the artisan farmers by working with them directly rather than through middle-men? (This improves world-economy and standard of living for many growers because many have been, and continue to be, unfairly treated by essential oil middlemen.)[17]
- Are your essential oils labeled as supplements? (This is a good thing.)
- Is *every* single batch of your prospective company's essential oils tested with rigorous internal *and* external testing? (Multiple-party testing is the only sure way to know exactly what you have in an essential oil. When you are researching essential oil testing, remember that third-party testing is more reliable than in-house testing. You may also want to ensure that testing is done on every batch of oil that comes in as opposed to randomly selected batches. Batches can differ greatly in chemical composition due to a variety of issues including natural reasons (rainfall, sunshine, and so on) and human intervention (time of harvest,

17 Caritas Czech Republic Mission in Aceh. "Support of Patchouli Growers in Aceh." Support of Patchouli Growers in Aceh -. AEDFF (Aceh Economic Development Financial Facility), 31 Aug. 2012. Web. 27 Apr. 2016. <http://svet.charita.cz/en/where-we-help/asia/indonesia/support-of-patchouli-growers-in-aceh/>.

time elapsed between harvest and distillation, additions or sub-
tractions to the oil, and so on).

Testing

Here are some important tests to watch for, which help determine
safety and efficacy of the essential oils tested:

But down deep, at the molecular heart of life, the trees and we are essentially identical.
—Carl Sagan

Gas Chromatography (GC): Gas Chromatography allows
chemical compounds to be separated, vaporized, and
analyzed. The essential oil compounds, once vaporized,
travel through a long column called a *gas chromatograph.*
Because each individual compound travels through the
column at a different rate, technicians are able to determine two things: which compounds are present and at
what levels.

Mass Spectrometry (MS): This test reveals the presence
of nonaromatic compounds (these can include heavy
metals, synthetics and chemicals to name a few) which
are too heavy to travel along the gas chromatograph,
and are undetectable in a GC. This test enables technicians to determine purity of the essential oil. The combination of gas chromatography and mass spectrometry
is often referred to as a *GC/MS.*

Fourier Transform Infrared Spectroscopy (FTIR) Scan:
The FTIR scan is a test that, when used in addition to the
GC/MS, can help ensure consistent standards as each
batch fits into the acceptable "chemical footprint" established by the company, and as it is measured against previous batches. In this test, a light is shown at the essential
oil sample and the amount of light absorbed (infrared

absorption) by the chemical constituents is measured and recorded.

Microbial Testing: The highest-quality essential oils will be tested to confirm the absence of bacteria, fungus, and mold. To test for these biohazards, samples from each batch of essential oils are applied to growing mediums in dishes, then allowed to incubate. At the end of the incubation period, each essential oil sample is analyzed for growth of microbes. This is an important test to do just before filling the bottles at the facility to ensure that no biohazards have been introduced to the oils at any point in the process from harvest and extraction to filling the bottles.

Organoleptic Testing: *Organoleptics* refers to qualities in a substance that relate to taste, sight, touch, and smell. Despite the fact that science plays a huge part in determining purity and potency of essential oils, they must also be pleasing and satisfy on a human-level. Experienced growers, harvesters, chemists, manufacturing engineers, and essential oil practitioners should monitor the quality of each batch as it passes through their stage of fulfillment until the end-user is able to enjoy a pure, potent and pleasing essential oil experience.

Let us permit nature to have her way. She understands her business better than we do.
—Michel de Montaigne

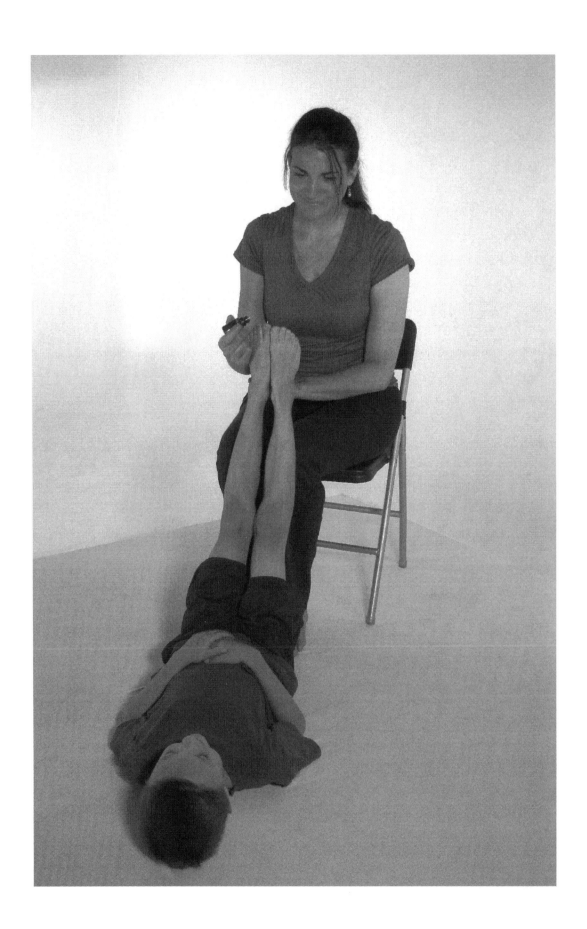

SECTION 9: THREE WAYS TO USE ESSENTIAL OILS

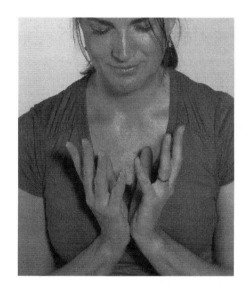

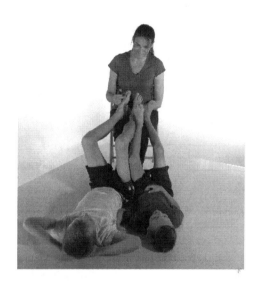

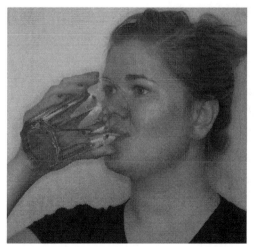

Aromatic

Using essential oils aromatically is the fastest way to get them into our system. When we breathe in oils, they enter our olfactory system,

The way to health is to have an aromatic bath and scented massage every day.
—Hippocrates

which is linked directly to the brain. Our brain is where we manage mood, trauma, memories and more. A complex and powerful interchange occurs as we breathe in oils. The simple summary is this: Essential oils can support our mood and outlook on life. They can help create an environment where we can better focus and concentrate on facts, goals, and/or creative ideas. They can provide support to our respiratory system (including lungs and sinuses). They can help reduce or even eliminate airborne pathogens. Because the olfactory system is the primary link between the central nervous system and the environment, inhaling essential oils directly benefits the central nervous system. Using oils aromatically while engaging in yoga allows us to create an ambience of our choosing as well as to promote a specific emotion during our yoga practice.

To use an oil aromatically, you can use a *diffuser,* which is a machine that disseminates essential oils into the air in a cool mist. Or, you can make your own personal diffuser by applying a drop of essential oil in the palm of one hand, rubbing your palms together, and cupping your nose with both hands while you inhale. Also, you can apply a drop of oil to a cotton ball to allow prolonged access to the aromatic properties of the oil.

Nature holds the key to our aesthetic, intellectual, cognitive and even spiritual satisfaction.
—E. O. Wilson

Topical

When we use pure and potent essential oils topically, the tiny molecular compounds in essential oils are quickly absorbed into the bloodstream. We can apply oils on location to calm minor skin irritations, to ease occasional stomach upset, to soothe minor burns and scrapes, and to help reduce tension, stress and worry. When we apply a drop of oil to the bottom of our feet, the oil is able to absorb quickly due to the larger pores on the bottom of the feet. The feet are the end of our lymphatic system—when we apply oils to the feet, the lymphatic system carries the microscopic compounds in essential oils to every cell and tissue of the body.

Note: Many people ask about when they should dilute essential oils with a carrier oil (such as fractionated coconut oil, olive oil, almond oil, and so on). If you consider that one or two drops is usually sufficient for an adult, it's a good idea to dilute oils for young children and babies or anyone with sensitive skin. Diluting a pure oil does not reduce the benefit of the oil; it reduces the possibility that the essential oils will cause sensitivity in the skin.

Important: If you apply a pure oil that produces a "burning" sensation, this means that your skin is sensitive to that oil. To soothe the skin immediately, apply a carrier oil, NOT water. Water and oil don't mix! Water drives the essential oil in faster, thus increasing the unwanted sensation. (If the oil you apply topically is not completely pure, there may be a chemical burn involved, and it may need to run its course before the skin is soothed.) For more information on safety guidelines, please see Section 12.

There is something of the marvelous in all things of nature.
—Aristotle

Internal

Please exercise caution when using essential oils internally; not all essential oils are sourced, extracted, or tested in a way that makes them safe for internal use. Follow bottle directions at all times.

When essential oils are 100 percent pure, and *when* they are approved for internal use (yes, there are some plants you should not use internally), they can support oral health, and healthy digestion and kidney function.

To use an oil internally, you can put a drop in water (make sure you use a glass, metal, or BPA-free plastic container), you can put drops under your tongue, or you can put drops in a capsule and swallow them like a vitamin.

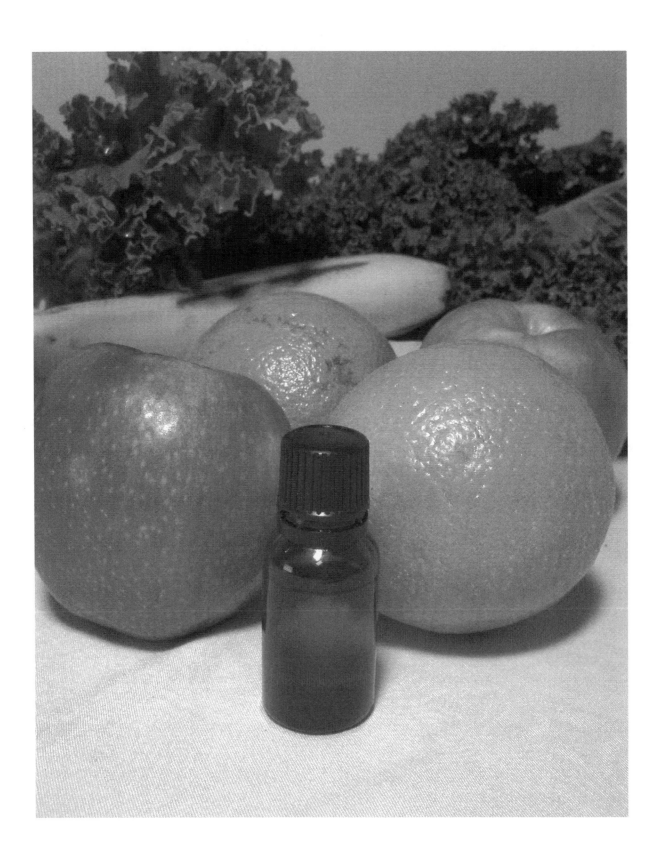

SECTION 10: ESSENTIAL OILS— CHEMICAL VERSUS NUTRITIONAL: WHAT ESSENTIAL OILS ARE NOT

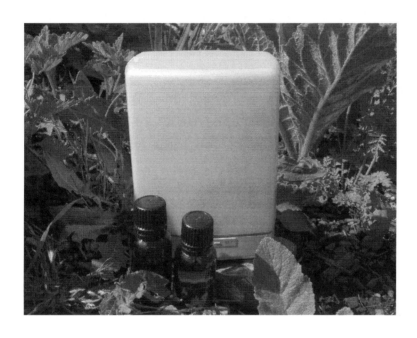

Health is the greatest gift, contentment the greatest wealth,
faithfulness the best relationship. —Buddha

It is important to recognize that essential oils work chemically within the body. They do *not* contain nutrients. Essential oils provide natural support as our body systems carry out their healthy functions.

It is important to nourish the body with bio-available, whole-food nutrients so that it can metabolize nutrients as usable fuel for the body. Getting the right amounts of nutrients helps you keep your Ph balance within the proper range and gives your cells the energy they need to function.

If you have been on a fast-food diet, or have been using or taking supplements that your body isn't absorbing properly, chances are that when you use essential oils, you won't receive their full benefit. You will most likely still receive some benefits, but your cells may not have the stamina and energy they need to work together with the essential oils to maximize their support to healthy body functions. Think about trying to drive to get your car's oil changed without enough gas in your tank; you can't optimize your car's performance without critical fuel.

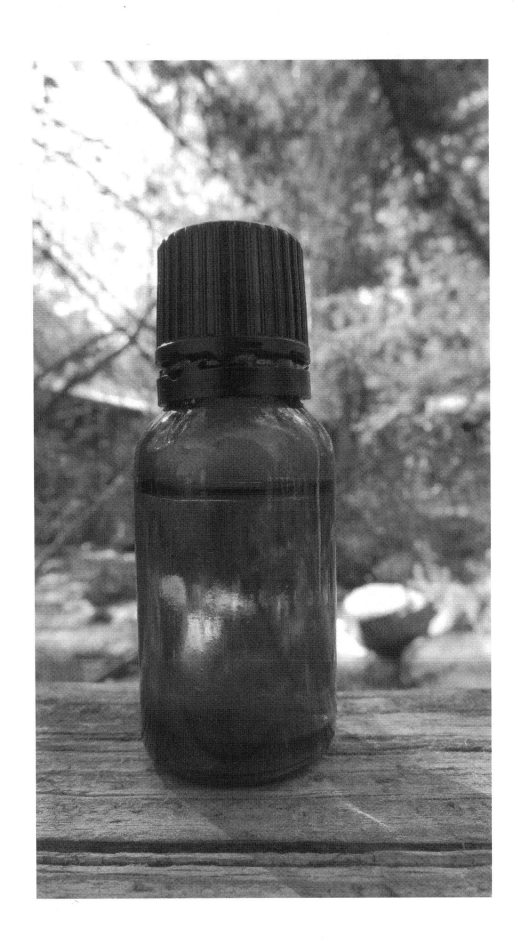

SECTION 11: ESSENTIAL OILS—SAFETY GUIDELINES

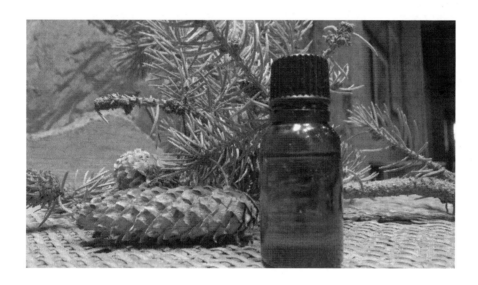

I want this day to be my fresh start. I want this to be the day I step out of my comfort zone and go somewhere new. —Jessi Kirby

After making sure that your essential oils are 100-percent pure, there are a few guidelines to follow that will help you have a positive oil experience.

First, never put oils in your eyes, ear canals, or inside your nose as these are sensitive tissues. If you would like to use essential oils to support eye wellness, you might consider diluting the essential oil with a carrier oil (such as fractionated coconut oil, olive oil, almond oil, and so on), applying a very small amount on the cheekbones or above the eyebrows, or using reflex points on the feet. When using oils topically to support ear and nose wellness, make sure the oils don't drip or get applied to the inner areas that can be so sensitive.

Second, realize that everyone has a different skin sensitivity. If the oil feels "hot" or uncomfortable on your skin, that oil probably has a high number of phenols. (*Phenols* are supportive to the immune system, but can cause some skin sensitivity.) To address the discomfort, simply apply a carrier oil directly on the area of concern and rub it in. You can also dilute an oil with carrier oil before applying it to avoid discomfort altogether.

Third, remember that with essential oils less is more. Only use a drop or two at a time, with consistency, to support your body systems as desired.

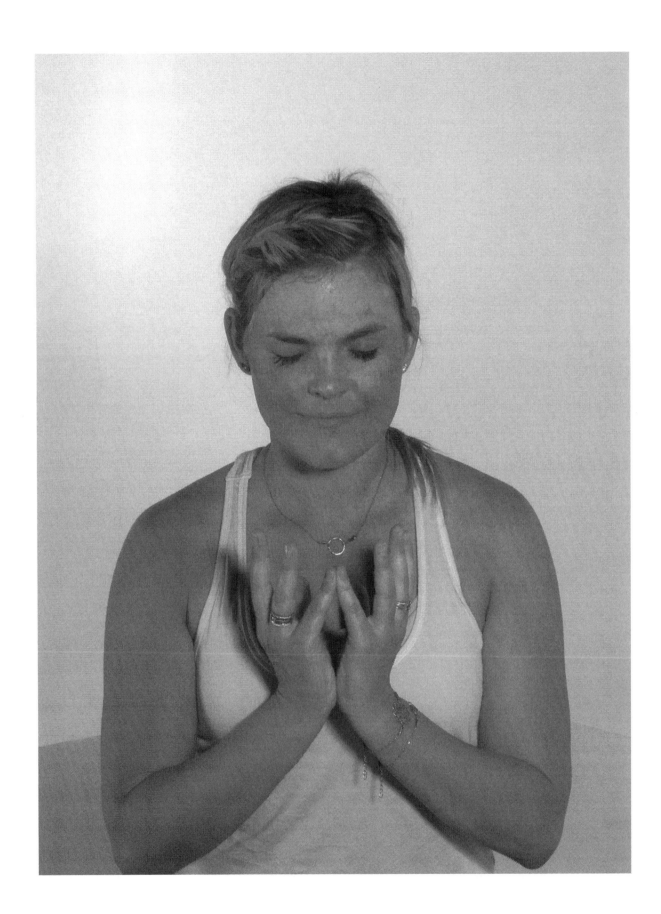

SECTION 12: HOW TO USE ESSENTIAL OILS WITH THE YOGA SEQUENCES IN THIS BOOK

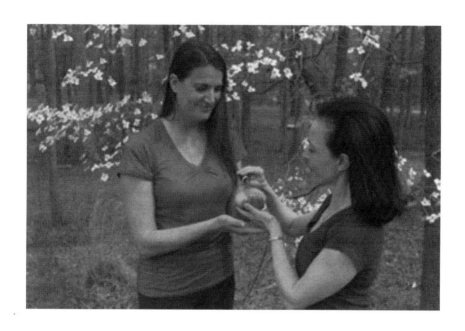

Take a quiet walk with Mother Nature. It will nurture your mind, body, and soul. —Anthony Douglas Williams

This book contains a series of Yoga sequences that were created with specific intentions to benefit body and soul. At the start of each sequence you will find a section with a list of suggested essential oils and/or essential oil blends for that sequence and a brief discussion of why those particular oils may be a powerful addition to your yoga experience.

You will also receive suggestions for how to apply or use the oils, and when to do so.

As you become more experienced and/or creative as you use essential oils, you can add or substitute oils as you see fit. The use of essential oils is a flexible practice—the goal is to resonate with the oil(s) you choose and enhance your experience as you support your well-being both physically and emotionally.

> **Note**: If your space and/or diffuser capacity is large, increase the amount of oil you use, with the same ratio, to better fit your space.

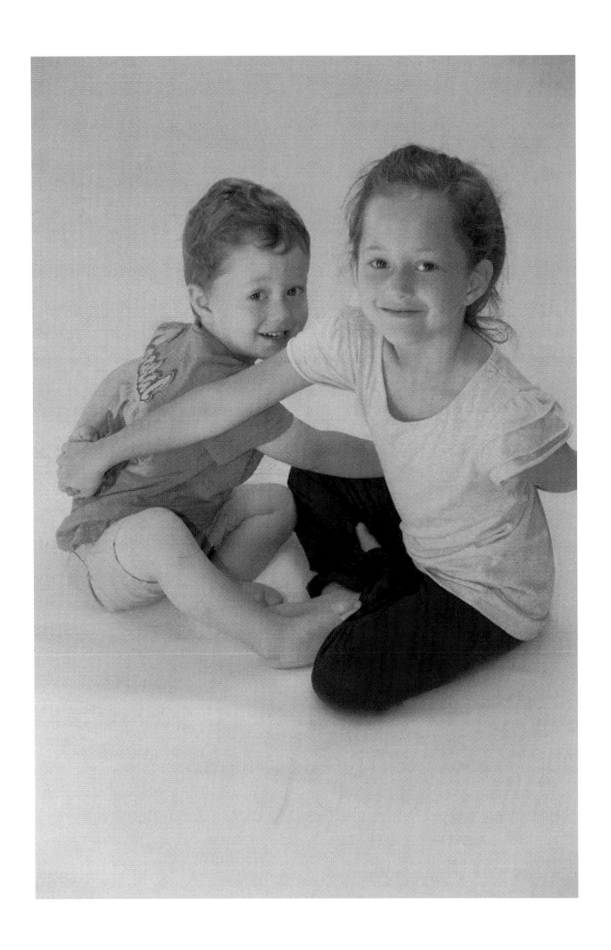

SECTION 13: ESSENTIAL YOGA PRACTICE BLOG

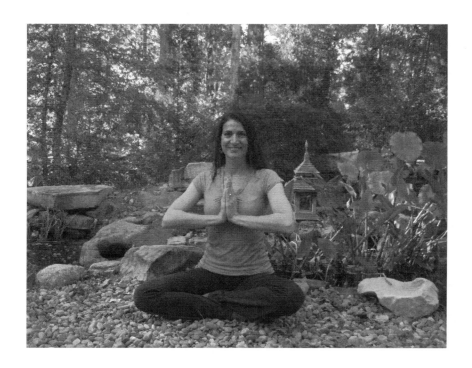

The earth has music for those who listen. —Shakespeare

You Are Invited!

We invite you to participate in our yoga blog, www.essentialyogapractice.com, which has been designed as a gathering space to connect essential oil and yoga enthusiasts. This is a place for beginning students and seasoned yogis alike. On this blog, http://www.essentialyogapractice.com/blog.html, you'll receive special insights, information, yoga, and essential oil tips—and of course, occasional gifts and prizes.

PART 3:
ESSENTIAL
YOGA PRACTICE
SEQUENCES

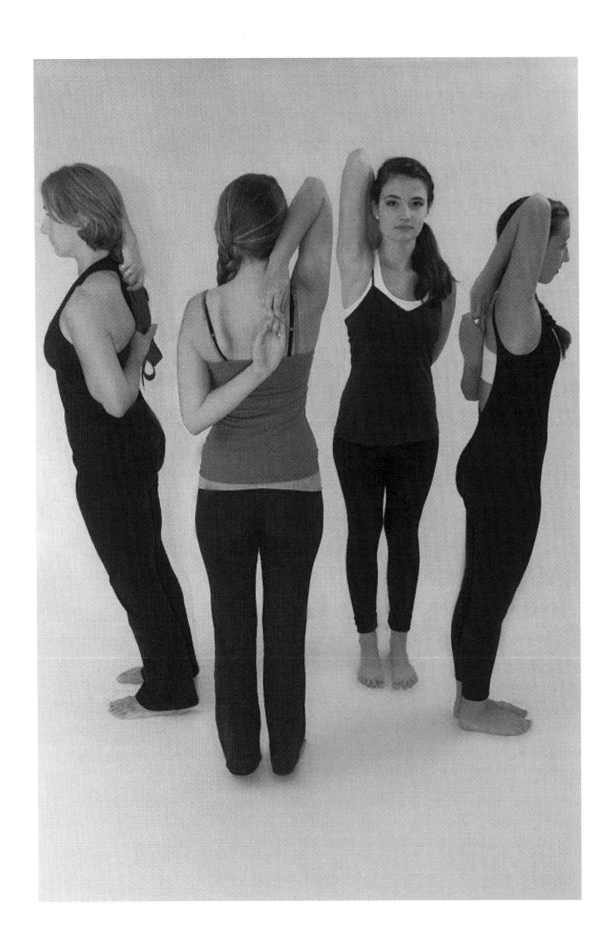

SEQUENCE 1: MORNING SEQUENCE

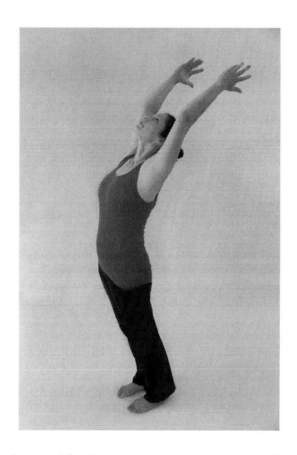

Today I choose life. Every morning when I wake up I can choose joy, happiness, negativity, pain...To feel the freedom that comes from being able to continue to make mistakes and choices—today I choose to feel life, not to deny my humanity but embrace it. —Kevyn Aucoin

Intention of the Morning Sequence

The intention of the morning sequence is to be energizing yet to provide clarity that will allow focus on what is ahead for the day. This means that we want to start with a grounding practice that will provide confidence for what we anticipate that day, with room to embrace un-expected events that unfold before us.

This yoga sequence is planned with poses to work all major muscle groups, moving the blood to wake up the body and stimulate the nervous system. When we start with standing poses, we are using our feet as they were designed—to be our foundation and to provide a grounding energy. The physiological aspect of standing poses is a direct message to the brain and nervous system to define which way is down, and to heighten awareness of the rebound energy of the ground. This rebound energy is our spring-board and we can think to use it physiologically, as well as emotionally.

Physically, we can put more internal action and mindfulness into the practice of each pose to maximize extension of the spine. Also, when we are more grounded energetically in our poses, the transitions from one pose to another will feel more solid. Emotionally, we will feel empowered by realizing our physical strength. In addition, increased endorphin levels add to the surge of feeling ready to take on the world.

> **Oil(s) to apply topically:** One drop each of grounding blend and massage blend the on bottom of each foot. After you rub the oil into the bottoms of your feet, cup your nose with your hands and breathe in the beautiful fragrance.

> **Oils to diffuse:** 1 drop geranium and 3 drops calming blend.

Grounding Blend_ This blend can include such oils as spruce, ho wood oil, frankincense, blue tansy, and blue chamomile in a base of fractionated coconut oil. An effective grounding blend helps you anchor—or center yourself—as it promotes tranquility and a sense of balance.

Human beings have layers of energy starting with systems on the inside of our bodies, and these energy layers expand outward several feet beyond our bodies. As we learn to be good stewards of these energy centers, we grow in strength and confidence. Our mood is enhanced. Our ability to connect with others and create/maintain positive relationships flourishes. Our influence and success grow from the inside out as we manage ourselves from the inside out.

Earlier in this book we discussed energy centers, chakras as well as the five sheaths of the body. Both are effected by and affect energy around and within you. The outermost sheath is the physical body. Let's start by considering the guidelines you use to govern your physical body. What do you eat? How much water do you drink? How much sleep do you get? Do you exercise enough? Do you stretch? Every decision we make regarding our physical bodies can either clear us—that is—allow energy and light to move more freely within us, or it can clog us by making it more difficult for energy to get around in us. The latter choice causes results that don't make us feel very good. We may feel sluggish, burned out, tired, apathetic, or worse.

A good grounding blend is typically comprised mostly of tree oils, or bass notes. Think of the strength and steadiness of trees—how they send roots deeply into the soil for solid anchoring. Tree oils support us as we strive to connect better to Mother Earth below us and open our minds to inspiration from our Higher Power above us. We become a conduit for the energy that flows all around us. What a beautiful way to start the day and open the pathway for additional essential oils.

Massage Blend
This blend can include such oils as cypress, marjoram, peppermint, basil, grapefruit. and lavender. The oils in the massage blend work together to help create flow and dissolve tension in the body. As we create flow and harmony physically, we open the possibility to create the same emotionally and mentally. Imagine what you can create each day

if you are intentional in your desire to balance and let ideas, creation, and resources flow to you and through you.

An added benefit of a good massage blend is that if you wake up with any particularly tense or tight areas, you can rub a drop of the massage blend into those specific areas to calm and soothe.

Geranium

I go to nature to be soothed and healed, and to have my senses put in order.
—John Burroughs

This is a beautifully fragrant oil that helps to calm nerves and lessen stress.

Calming Blend

This blend can include oils such as lavender, sweet marjoram, Roman chamomile, ylang ylang, sandalwood, and vanilla absolute bean extract. The oils in a calming blend work together to create a sense of calming and renewing. A calming blend promotes relaxation, lessens tension, and reduces worry and stress. Starting the day from a space of emotional peace and calm helps us set a beautiful tone.

Sequence Instructions:

Props needed: Yoga mat, two blocks, one strap, yoga blanket, eye pillow (optional)

Practice preparation: Come to the front end of your mat, put a few drops of your essential oils in your palm, and rub your hands together. Bring your hands together in Anjali mudra, keeping the thumbs and pinky fingers together. Spread the fingers wide to create your personal diffuser. Rest your thumbs against your chest, drop your chin to your chest, and breathe. If the aroma is too strong, adjust your personal diffuser to be less open.

Transition your hand position to the "prayer position," Anjali Mudra, or Namaskarasana, as some refer to this position, in front of your heart. Use this time to create an intention for your practice today. It can be a meditation, prayer, mantra, word, or an idea that you want to manifest or support in your life.

Suggested length of time in each pose: Sun Salute poses—transition with either an inhalation or an exhalation in each pose as explained in each pose description, below. For the rest of the poses, stay 20-40 seconds in each. That is the general recommendation for beginners. Intermediate yogis aim to build more time and resilience in a pose, but more importantly, to gain a deeper awareness of both the physical and the emotional components of each pose.

Insights about this sequence: Each pose (or series of poses) in this sequence is separated by capital letters in the outline form below.

You'll find the first sequence, Surya Namaskar—also known as Sun Salute—in Section A, below. Once you are familiar with Surya Namaskar, with consistent practice, you will build awareness as well as strength. Then you can use it as a standalone practice for a greater length of time either by adding more repetitions or by staying longer in each pose.

The sequence is designed to be done at least twice, once with the right leg leading, and the second time with the left leg leading. It is not uncommon for seasoned yogis to build up to 12 sets (6 reps for each side to lead, alternating right and left each time) and use only a Sun Salutation as a workout for the hour.

There are many variations on a Sun Salute. Once you have memorized the sequence, you will be surprised at the intuition of your body and the memory of your yoga body from your general practice, as to what poses you are inclined to sandwich into a Sun Salutation, still doing one set led with the right leg, and one set led with the left leg. Initially, try to move from one pose to another in the Sun Salute using the length of a long inhalation or a long exhalation to determine the amount of time you stay before transitioning to the next pose. Once you finish using a Sun Salute warm-up, in the rest of this sequence, try to stay 20–40 seconds in each pose if you are a beginner. Remember that all actions in yoga are light and in all poses, each limb has a job so that the work in the body becomes comprehensive through counterbalancing actions which create balance and thus, create safety. There should not be any straining.

You can use just the Sun Salute if you just have a short amount of time, but if you have time for more, *please follow the entire sequence in the order shown below for safety*. The placement of each pose in the sequence is designed to provide a preparation or a recovery that will, in turn, allow success and safety in the pose that follows.

Morning Sequence
A. Surya Namaskar—Sun Salute
1. Tadasana, Mountain Pose

- Come to the front end of the mat and stand with feet together unless knees come together first.
- Press down the big toe mounds and take weight off the other eight toes. Lift both the inner and outer arches of the feet.
- Lift with the muscles of the front body and ground with the muscles of the back body. Bring your awareness to lifting the kneecaps, lifting the pelvic

floor, drawing the navel to the spine, lifting the sternum, and broadening the collarbones while letting the tailbone length-en downward, allowing the shoulder blades to slide down, and draw both the inner and outer thighs back. All of this might seem a bit too much to think about at first, but as you become a seasoned yogi, you will find that you balance the detail of all of these very light actions well, and are ready to refine your pose more.

Yoga means addi-tion—addition of energy, strength and beauty to body, mind and soul.
— Amit Ray

- Bring your hands to your heart in Namaskarasana and take a few breaths to focus on your intention.

2. Urdhva Hastasana, Volcano Pose

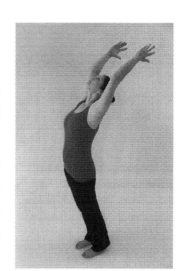

- From Mountain Pose, inhale and lift up arms overhead, elbows straight, and aim to align elbows with the ears.
- Imagine your shoulderblades want to wrap around to the sides of the ribcage, creating more space between them. Inhale and broaden the ribcage even more, from within, using your breath.
- Reach down to reachup, lifting the ribs off the hips.

3. Uttanasana, Standing Forward Bend

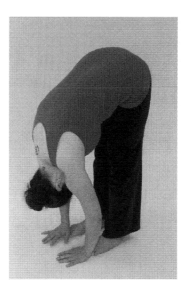

- Exhale and fold from the hips, letting head hang while continuing to length-en the front of the spine. If your fold is deep, look up to the belly. The arms can hang, or you can catch hold of the big toes, ankles, or back of the calf to draw yourself deeper into the fold.

- Microbend the knees, reach down with the inner heels, and lift with the sitting bones. This will protect the sacroiliac spine.

4. Extended Standing Forward Bend

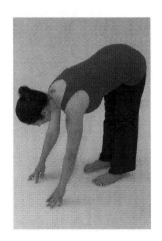

- Inhale and extend the spine. Either place hands at the shins, and press lightly back, or place fingertips at the floor. Lightly press down and forward as you gaze ahead to the floor a few feet ahead. The primary action here is extension of the front of the spine. Think "leading with the heart."

5. Lunge, Right Leg Back

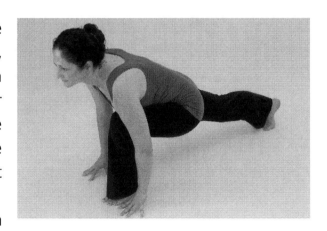

- Exhale and lunge back the right leg, placing hands on the floor, shoulder width apart, one hand on each side of the left foot, front knee at 90 degrees.
- Use the left arm pressing into the left leg/inner knee and resist with the leg. Inhale and lengthen from the back inner heel through to the crown of the head, allowing the front spine to lengthen.

6. High Plank

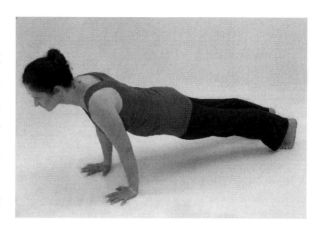

- Exhale and step back the left leg to arrive in Plank. If you cannot bear your body weight on the hands and toes while holding the body straight from the heels to the head, bend in the knees and rest the shins on the floor. Inhale, broaden the collarbones while extending the front spine forward and reaching into the inner heels.

7. Chatarangua, Push Up Pose

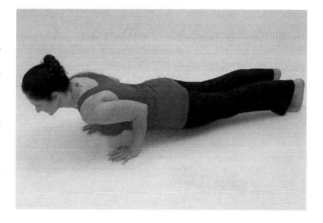

- Exhale and bend the elbows, slowly lowering the body toward the floor, keeping the elbows close to the rib cage.
- Pause with elbows at 90 degrees and over wrists, core muscles engaged. Then continue toward the floor, resting the weight of the body on the floor. If this is too much at first, include bending in the knees, resting them first at the floor.

8. Urdhva Mukha Svanasana, Upward Facing Dog

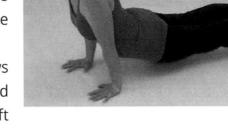

- Inhale and keeping the legs/hips resting on the floor, press the hands into the floor.
- Straighten the elbows any amount, spread the collarbones, lift the sternum, and look upwards.

9. Adho Mukha Svanasana, Downward Facing Dog

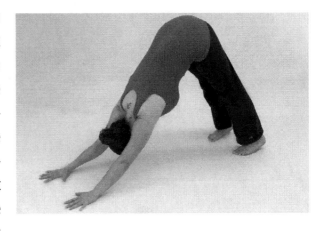

- Exhale and begin to shift the hips back and up, folding from the hips. Allow the head to hang,, gazing back toward the knees. The abdominals will contract to help provide the movement of this transition.
- Press into the heels of the hands—more at the thumb side.
- Roll the shoulders open, creating space across the shoulder blades, and draw up the head of the humerus (the upper arm) into the shoulder joint.

- Though your heels are not touching the floor, reach into the inner heels.
- Let the head hang so that the neck will release.
- Allow slow deep breathing to help create space between the shoulder blades

10. Lunge, Right Leg Forward

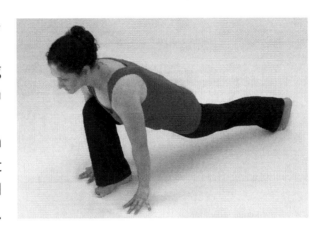

- Inhale, lift your head, look ahead.
- Lunge the right leg forward to between the hands.
- Use the right arm pressing into the right inner leg/knee and resist with the leg. Inhale and lengthen from the back inner heel through to the crown of the head, allowing the front spine to lengthen.
- Exhale, and step the back leg to the front leg.

11. Extended Standing Forward Bend

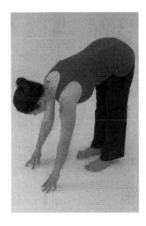

- Inhale, and extend the spine, following the same actions as above in #4.

12. Uttanasana, Standing Forward Bend

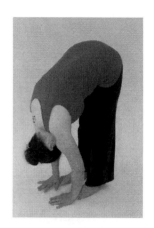

- Exhale, and fold down, hanging the head and looking up to the navel.
- Microbend the knees, reach down with the inner heels, and lift with the sitting bones. This will protect the sacroiliac spine.

13. Utkatasana, Powerful Pose

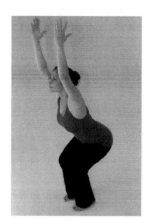

- Inhale, and swing up both arms as you pause in a squat, and begin to unfold.
- Lift up the ribs—away from the hips.

14. Urdhva Hastasana, Volcano Pose

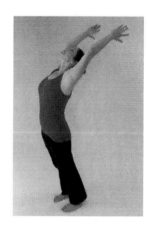

- Continue the inhale, and come all the way up, following the cues from above, as in #2.
- Inhale, lift your gaze to look up to your hands and invite a small backbend into the upper ribcage.

15. Tadasana, Mountain Pose

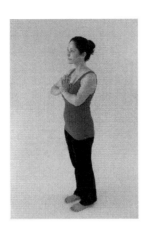

- Exhale, and return hands to the heart in prayer.
- Take a few breaths before beginning again to notice the difference in initiating with the right side.

16. Repeat the Sun Salute sequence, leading with the left leg on poses #5 and #10.

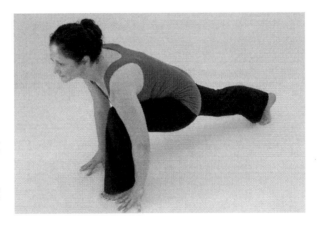

- Coming again to the end of the Sun Salute, stand and reflect inward. Notice the return of balance to the body having completed the sequence with the left side leading. Remind yourself of the intention of your practice for today.

B. Parivrtta Parsvakonasana—Revolved Side Angle Pose

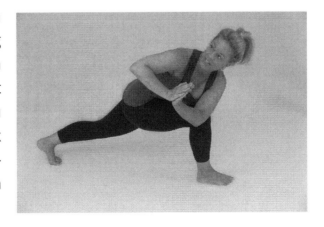

- Stand sideways on your mat, stepping feet wide, and turn the right foot out 90 degrees. As you pivot off the back leg, turning the upper body to face in the direction of the right foot, make sure you are not "walking the tight rope."

- Bend the right knee, and fold from the hips to come into a lunge with the right foot forward between the hands, left leg back. If it is too difficult to put your hands on the floor, on either side of the front foot, place each hand on a yoga block, or on the seat of a chair in front of you, if you need to be higher. Front leg is with knee bent to 90 degrees; back leg is straight.
- Extend right arm forward so that it follows the line of the back leg, palm facing down, hand higher than the head.
- Using the leverage of the left hand at the floor, block or chair below, turn the torso/rib cage to the right, looking underneath the right armpit toward the wall/ceiling behind you.
- Breathe deeply and with an inhale, begin slowly to come out of this pose sending both arms reaching forward.
- Stay another breath or two to challenge and build the strength of the front leg/hip. Keep the legs firm and steady.
- Inhale and come unfolding to an upright position, to the next pose, Warrior I.

C. Virabhadrasana I—Warrior I

- Right leg is forward with front knee bent to ninety degrees if possible and, if protecting a knee issue, do not bend as deeply.
- Left leg is back with leg straight.
- Front foot is flat on the floor, and the back foot for beginners is also flat to ensure more steady grounding.
- For those wanting a balancing challenge, try to send the back leg further back and stay at the ball of the foot—all toes facing forward.
- Lift up the arms overhead to help lift the rib cage.

- If back foot is down, reach down into the outer back heel and up into the fingertips. If back foot it with heel lifted, reach into inner back heel instead.
- Breathe fully and deeply. Hip flexors will lengthen accordingly. Notice how your breath travels into all three lobes of the lungs (frontal, lateral, and posterior).
- Draw the front lower ribs to the back ribs to engage the core.
- Then, turn to the side and walk or hop the feet together to center. Repeat these two poses linked together with the left leg leading.

D. Garudasana—Eagle Pose

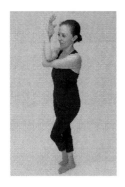 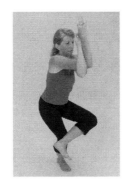 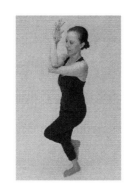

- Stand on the left leg and cross the right leg over the left, propping ball of the right foot against the floor.
- Push into both feet and keep the hips even from the floor, thus not hiking one hip out to the side or up.
- Seasoned students will either place the right ankle at the left knee and sit into the pose as in Utkatasana (chair pose) or wrap the right leg around the left.
- Cross the left elbow over the right and wrap the arms to include the hands while holding the elbows at approximately shoulder height. Press the elbows lightly into each other to create space between the shoulder blades. Maintaining the alignment, reach elbows forward with only internal action. Inhale and allow the

deep breath to continue increasing the space between the shoulder blades.

- Exhale, reach down into both legs, and use the rebound energy to lift the ribs off the hips. Stay an additional couple of breaths and inhale to come out of the pose, opening the arms wide to engage the opposing muscles of the shoulder.

- Repeat with the left foot crossed and propped over the right and the right elbow crossed over the left elbow.

- If you cannot wrap the hands, bring both hands and elbows together, and follow the same cues as above, or wrap and hug the arms around the body.

E. Standing Gomukhasana—Cow Face Pose

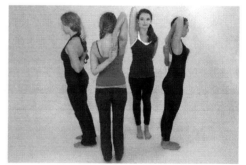

- Place the yoga strap over your right shoulder so that one end hangs down the front of the body, and the other end hangs down the back of the body.

- Begin by taking the right hand to the strap at the top of the shoulder and, following the strap, reach as far back as you can with the right hand sliding down the back, elbow pointing toward the ceiling—not out to the side.

- Take the left hand from below at the back, find the strap, and walk the left hand up the back/strap as far as possible without straining either shoulder. If you can hook three fingers, you can ignore the strap. Otherwise, hold the strap with both hands in a tugging fashion.

- As you stand with feet hip-width apart, reach into the inner heels, lengthen the tailbone down, lift the pelvic floor and the pit of the abdomen.

- Draw the front ribs to the back ribs to keep the lower back from hyperextending. Stay for a few deep breaths here.

- Inhale to come out of the pose and do the other side.

F. Supta Padangusthasana I, II, III—Reclined Hand to Big Toe I, II, III

1. Supta Padangusthasana I

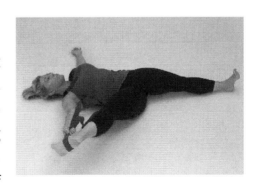

- Lying on the mat, take the right leg, knee straight, up toward the ceiling, and keep the left leg at the floor.
- Place the strap at the ball of the right foot, and hold the strap with one or both arms, elbows straight. If your head drops back (tight neck/shoulders), prop the head up with a folded blanket or towel so that the neck is parallel to the floor.
- Shoulder blades slide down the back body to help "hold the reigns" in this pose.
- Flex the bottom foot, and reach into the inner heels of both feet.
- Lengthen the tailbone away from the head.
- Draw in the pit of the abdomen.
- Anchor the left inner thigh toward the floor while (primary action) sending the right hip (internal action) away from the ribs, toward the left heel.

2. Supta Padangusthasana II

- Take the straps in the right hand and keeping the pelvis level with the floor, drop the right leg to the right, reaching the left arm along the floor to the left, to oppose the pull of the right leg. Anchor with the left side of the pelvis.

115

- Stay a few breaths and work into all four limbs. Use the leverage of all the actions to maintain your longest spine.
- Exhale to bring the leg back to center.

3. Supta Padangusthasana III

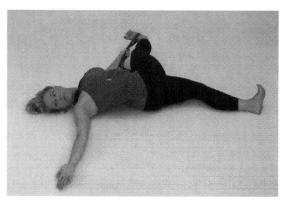

- Inhale and switch the straps into the left hand.
- Take the right leg across the midline toward the left, and choose between two options: For someone with a weak or compromised lower back, take the right leg across only until the right foot lines up with the left shoulder, and the pelvis stays even with the floor. Otherwise, take the leg across as far as possible while keeping the shoulders even with the floor. Here, the pelvis should tip to the left. Continue to reach the right sitting bone away from the head.
- The right arm reaches out to the right, to counterbalance the right leg..

G. Sukhasana Twist—Happy Pose Twist

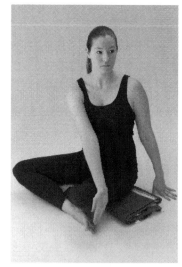

- Sit on a folded yoga blanket, legs crossed. The height of the blanket should allow the height of the knees to be even with the level of the hip bones.
- Turning to the left, place the right hand on the outer left knee—palm away—and place the left hand on the floor or on a block behind the left hip.

- The left hand pushes down at the floor to help extend the spine upward; both hands help equally to guide the twist. Stay for a few breaths.
- Inhale to come out of the pose.
- Exhale to turn toward the right side. Repeat the pose.

H. Pranayama I—Meditation Pose with Viloma I Breath Work

This elementary setup for meditation is very traditional as is the breathing exercise that goes along with it. One advantage of the physical practice of yoga is to strengthen and condition the body—particularly the spine—to be able to sit in meditation for 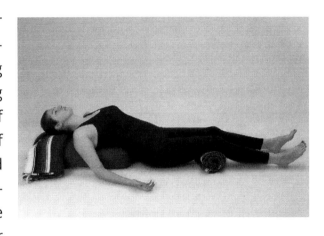 significant periods of time. For beginners, the back gets tired quickly, so this supported, reclined position is often used to learn to build time in meditation.

- Set a yoga bolster lengthwise with the mat and place a folded blanket on top of one end. This will serve as your "pillow" to support the neck and head. Sit at the other end of the bolster and recline so that you are lying with the back and rib cage supported. Roll up another blanket and place it under the knees. Rest with head centered and arms beside you, palms up.
- To begin the breathing exercise, focus on lengthening both the inhalation and the exhalation. Initially, you may feel the need to take a few normal shorter breaths. As soon as you can, return to lengthening the breath. Then, begin to think of the torso as a "funnel" with the lower part being your pubic bone and the upper open part being your collar bones/shoulders.

- Your next breaths will be divided into three sections. Inhale slowly and relax your abdomen inviting the breath to fill the lower part of the funnel. Continue the deep breath, and notice how you can direct this second part to broadening the rib cage near the floating ribs. Continue the inhalation, taking as deep a breath as you can. Notice how your breath feels as if it travels up into your shoulders.

- Once you are ready to exhale, let the bottom of the funnel empty first, dropping the belly, and then let the rest of the breath go, emptying the rib cage from the top to the middle. If you need a few shorter, "regular" breaths, honor that. Then, return to this three-part breathing exercise.

- Once you no longer need the few shorter breaths, then you are ready to add some "retention." Between each section and at the top of the breath, pause for a second or two and begin to notice—especially at the top of the breath—how your body/rib cage seems to want to continue to expand even when you are not taking in more air. These areas of retention will also serve as places to increase your internal awareness.

- Once you are finished with this pranayama exercise, remain in this supported position for meditation and notice the body's continued use of slow deep breathing.

This wonderful pranayama exercise is a great tool to use to wake up the diaphragm and intercostal muscles, oxygenate the body, build lung capacity, and deter the mind from "racing" on to next things in the thought process. At the end of your meditation time, bring back your focus to your intention and resolve to keep it for the rest of your day.

Morning Sequence at-a-Glance

A. Sun Salute:

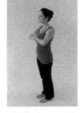 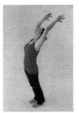 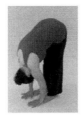 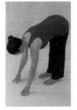 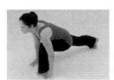

A1. Tadasana / Mountain Pose | A2. Urdhva Hastasana / Volcano Pose | A3. Uttanasana / Standing Forward Bend | A4. Extended Standing Forward Bend | A5. Lunge Right Leg Back

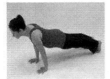 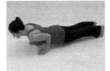 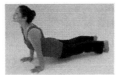 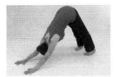 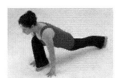

A6. High Plank | A7. Chatarangua / Push Up Pose | A8. Urdhva Mukha Svanasana / Upward Facing Dog | A9. Adho Mukha Svanasana / Downward Facing Dog | A10. Lunge Right Leg Forward

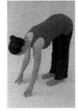 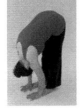 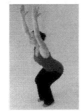 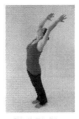 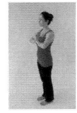 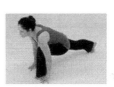

A11. Extended Standing Forward Bend | A12. Uttanasana / Standing Forward Bend | A13. Utkatasana / Chair Pose | A14. Urdhva Hastasana / Volcano Pose | A15. Tadasana / Mountain Pose | **A16. Repeat Sun Salute sequence** Leading with left leg on 5th & 10th poses.

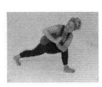 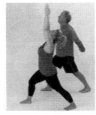 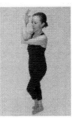 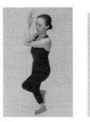

B. Parivrtta Parsvakonasana / Revolved Side Angle Pose | C. Virabhadrasana I / Warrior I | D. Garudasana / Eagle Pose Beginning – Intermediate - Advanced | E. Standing Gomukhasana / Cow Face Pose

 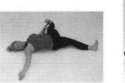 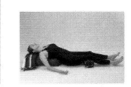

F. Supta Padangusthasana I, II & III / Hand to Big Toe Pose I, II & III | G. Sukhasana Twist / Happy Pose Twist | H. Pranayama I / Meditation Pose with Viloma I Breath Work

119

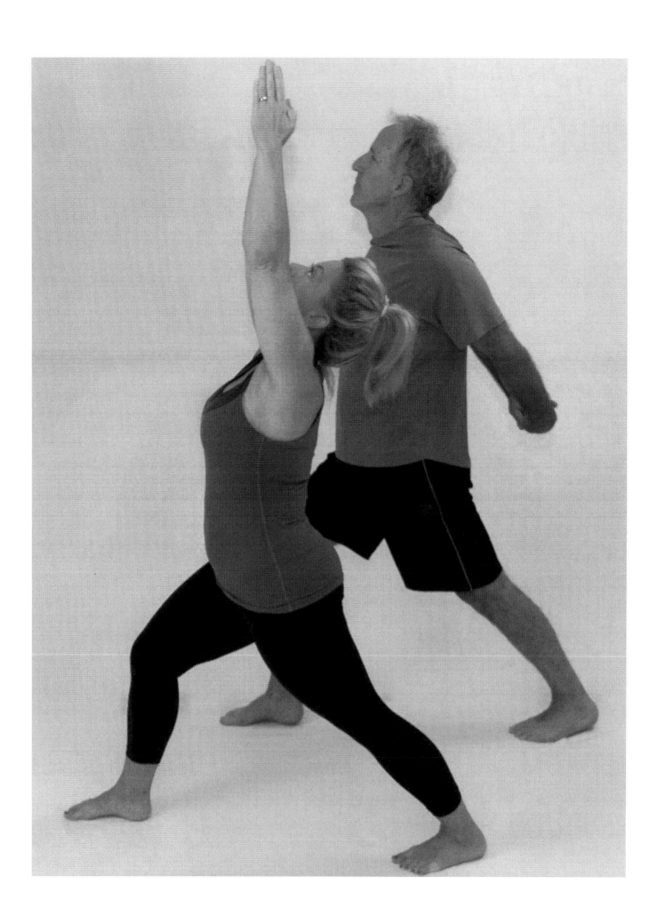

SEQUENCE 2: STRENGTHENING SEQUENCE

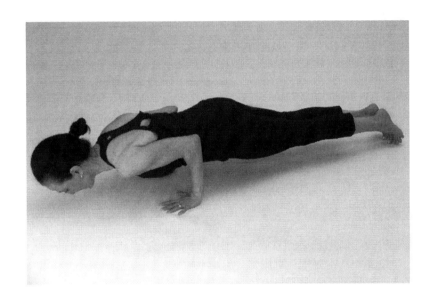

If I'm losing balance in a pose, I stretch higher and God reaches down to steady me. It works every time, and not just in yoga. —T. Guillemets

Intention of the Strengthening Sequence

The intention of the strengthening sequence is to build resilience in body, mind, and spirit. We are built to move, and we need to move daily. When we do not move, not only do the muscles atrophy, but their relationship with joint structure and innervation from the nervous system is also compromised. In addition, hormonal stimulation is diminished.

When we put our muscles through a workout intended to build strength, we are also using our strength to create the movement. We get to both see and feel ourselves being strong, not just managing, but mastering the work performed. Emotionally, this has an empowering effect. For those with compromised bodies, practicing with care to adjust for injuries, watching the building of strength in the body helps with learning to trust the body again. Cells regenerate with muscle memory of stimulation. Thus, overall health and wellness improves with consistent daily exercise and movement. Movement designed to build strength physically can only translate to ensuring our sense of readiness to live our purpose.

> **Oil(s) to apply topically:** 1 drop each of bergamot and ginger. Apply over the heart, and rub in a clockwise motion for ten seconds each. (**Note:** Ginger is an oil that some may find sensitive on the skin. Either dilute it prior to application, or have a carrier oil handy to apply in case if discomfort.) Also apply a drop of bergamot to the area just above your belly button and rub in a clockwise motion (as if the front side of your body is the face of a clock). After applying the oils, cup your nose with your hands and breathe in the beautiful fragrance.

> **Oils to diffuse:** 1 drop of cilantro and 1 drop calming blend. (**Note:** Cilantro has a deep, rich aroma. If its aroma is too strong for you, soften the blend by using 1 drop frankincense instead. Clary sage, cypress, and cinnamon are other oils that are ideal to use in conjunction with this sequence.

Bergamot

This is a citrus oil that has a subtle and tangy fragrance. It helps reduce tension and stress and lessen sad or anxious feelings. As we strive to develop strength in our physical bodies, most of us recognize the importance of strengthening our *core*—that place within the trunk of our body that anchors and centers the actions and stability of our extremities.

On a parallel plane, we must strengthen our emotional core if we wish truly to have strength. Interestingly, the third chakra—or energy center—that represents how we value ourselves is found in the area that we associate with our physical core. Use bergamot on your heart and core to keep your intention aligned with strengthening the very essence of yourself while realizing your value and uniqueness. Consider how your unique gifts and qualities—once developed and honed—can bless and touch those around you in a way that can come only from you. Commit to develop the strength that will keep you anchored in Mother Earth for support as you seek to support others.

Ginger

Historically, ginger has been used to support healthy digestion as well as ease occasional indigestion and nausea. It has a hot, earthy, spicy, and sweet aroma that has added zest and flavor to sweet and savory dishes around the world. As this beautiful oil supports healthy physical digestion, think also about your "emotional digestion," or how you perceive or interpret the events around you.

Whether we like it or not, our current circumstances are the result of our past actions. The present is the only moment of true power we have because it is the only moment we can choose to take full advantage of. The choices we make today impact what our future looks like.

Breathe in and appreciate the hot, spicy sweet aroma of ginger, and choose to seize the day. Fill your heart with courage to take responsibility for every facet of your life. Only when you choose to let go of blame, regret, and resentment can you develop that core of strength you were meant to have always. You are a creator. What do you choose to do with your power?

Cilantro

Cilantro is a powerful cleanser and detoxifier. It is rich in antioxidants known to protect the body's cells from oxidative stress. It promotes healthy digestion and adds a fresh, herbal aroma to any essential oil blend when diffused.

When we have experiences that we interpret negatively, we in turn create negative emotions appropriate to our reaction to the event. We might feel sadness, hurt, anger, fear, or guilt. Negative emotions are made of energy that vibrate on a low frequency, and we send all that low vibration into our bodies.

Very few of us do an adequate job of clearing negative emotions as we experience them. The result is that we store negative emotion over long periods of time, sometimes even years. Eventually, this negative energy takes a toll on our bodies by creating weaknesses that manifest in specific organs and/or systems. (If you'd like to learn more about this topic, read Louise Hay's book *You Can Heal Your Life*.)

As you perform the strengthening sequence and diffuse the fresh, herbal aroma of cilantro, we invite you to let go of what is no longer serving you. Instead, focus on positive strength. Intentionally raise the frequency, or vibration, that you live by.

The art of healing comes from nature and not from the physician. Therefore, the physician must start from nature with an open mind.
—Paracelsus

Calming Blend

This blend can include oils such as lavender, sweet marjoram, Roman chamomile, ylang ylang, sandalwood, and vanilla absolute bean extract. The oils in a calming blend work together to create a sense of calming and renewing. A calming blend promotes relaxation, lessens tension, and reduces worry and stress. Starting the day—or returning to a space of emotional peace and calm any time during the day—helps us set a beautiful tone for our lives intentionally. Marianne Williamson said,

Our deepest fear is not that we are inadequate. Our deepest fear is that we are powerful beyond measure. It is our light, not our darkness that most frightens us. We ask ourselves, Who am I to be brilliant, gorgeous, talented, and fabulous? Actually, who are you not to be? You are a child of God. Your playing small does not serve the world. There is nothing enlightened about shrinking so that other people will not feel insecure around you. We are all meant to shine, as children do. We were born to make manifest the glory of God that is within us. It is not just in some of us; it is in everyone and as we let our own light shine, we unconsciously give others permission to do the same. As we are liberated from our own fear, our presence automatically liberates others.[18]

It takes work to detoxify ourselves emotionally so we can show up in the strength of our power. A good calming blend is the perfect companion to the cleansing effects of cilantro to calm the mind, relax the body, and soothe the soul when we are feeling vulnerable and emotional from life's daily stressors. Yoga is the perfect companion to these oils because it reminds us that there is great power in being still, and that it's OK to lean on others as we increase our personal fortitude. Yoga practice coupled with pure, potent essential oils helps create an environment where toxic release is facilitated and strength is restored.

Sequence Instructions:

Props needed: Yoga mat, two blocks, one strap, yoga blanket.

---

18   *A Return to Love: Reflections on the Principles of "A Course in Miracles,"* HarperCollins; New York; Ch. 7, Section 3 (1992) p. 190

Practice preparation: Come to the front end of your mat after putting 1–2 drops of essential oils in your hands, bring your hands together in Anjali mudra. Keep the thumbs and pinky fingers together, and spread the fingers wide to create your personal diffuser. Rest your thumbs against your chest, drop your chin to your chest, and breathe. Root the inner heels to the floor, and reach up through the crown of the head. Feel the broadening of your rib cage. Resolve to use the rebound energy from your reach into the earth to support the intention of your practice.

Suggested length of time in each pose: Beginning yogis: 20–40 seconds, Intemediate/advanced yogis: 40–60 seconds. (**Note**: Considering that this sequence aims to build strength and resilience, don't be surprised if you pass through the beginning stage to the intermediate stage very quickly.)

Insights about this sequence: The Warrior Sequence (Section A) makes for a great warm-up on its own and is designed to both open up and strengthen the hips. Considering that the hips are the base of the spine, attention to creating balance in the pelvis, with regard to strength and flexibility, means that the rest of the frame (particularly the structure of the spine and rib cage) will not have to compensate for imbalance. Interestingly enough, imbalance in the hips can be either the cause or result of structural imbalances in the legs and feet. No matter what currently exists regarding back, shoulder, or neck issues, attention to aligning and balancing the hips is in order for everyone.

In addition, warrior poses are used to invoke a sense of readiness, and holding a warrior pose is an opportunity to clarify thinking while anticipating what comes next. Thus, warrior poses are often placed before other more

The nature of yoga is to shine the light of awareness into the darkest corners of the body.
— Jason Crandell

intricate poses to build on this process. Beginning to use this idea "off the mat" becomes quite valuable in thinking well on your feet in our often fast paced world.

Strengthening Sequence

A. Warrior Sequence
1. Virabhadrasana I—Warrior I

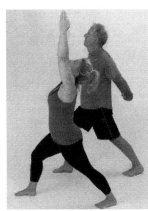

- Stand with the right leg well forward, right knee bent, keeping the left leg straight, left foot turned somewhat forward.
- Lift the arms up and aim to have shoulders at the ears.
- Keeping both feet/heels anchored, reach down into the outer back heel, and use the rebound energy to reach up into the fingertips, lifting the rib cage as the primary action.
- To enhance the hip flexor release, draw the navel to the spine and the front ribs toward the back ribs.
- Stay for three to five breaths.
- Lifting to the ball of the left foot, take the arms wide, pivot to the left, and plant the left foot flat, arriving in the next pose.

2. Virabhadrasana II—Warrior II

- Once you turn to the left side, adjust your feet to "walking the tightrope" aiming to be all on one plane.

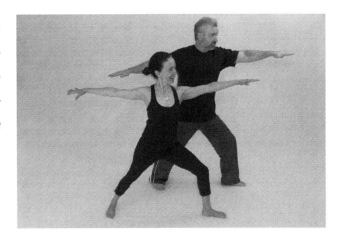

- The front, right leg is still bent and the back leg with foot slightly pigeon-toed is still straight.
- The arms, held at shoulder height, have two opposing actions: all the muscles engage lightly as if to hug the bones, while at the same time, try to grow the wingspan.
- Turn your head to look over the right hand.
- Invite the hips to open while firming the legs to the floor.
- Lift the pelvic floor and draw the navel to the spine.
- Stand at your tallest spine and stay three to five breaths.
- Then lift up to the ball of the left foot, begin to pivot off the back foot, and return to facing forward, taking the arms up and returning to your Warrior I.

3. Warrior I

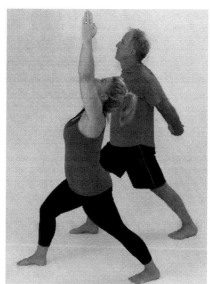

- If you can stay on the ball of the foot here, you have a bit more of a challenge to balance, thus enhancing that ability in your body. You can try to square the hips with the front end of your mat here.
- Though the back heel is off the floor, still reach into the inner back heel, and lift the rib cage as you reach into the fingertips.
- After three to five breaths, fold forward from the hips—reaching the arms forward—and come to balancing on the right leg. You are arriving in the next pose.

4. Virabhadrasana III—Warrior III

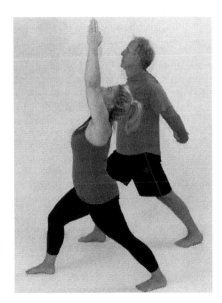

- Straighten the right leg—lifting the left leg straight back behind—and reach into both inner heels, making sure the back foot is flexed.
- While the arms reach forward to oppose the reach of the leg back, find a comfortable challenge in dropping the left hip, aiming to square the hips with the floor.
- Once you are here for three to five breaths, lift the arms to drop the back leg.
- Once again, arrive in Warrior I—this time planting your back foot well behind you.

5. Warrior I

- Reclaiming the actions of your Warrior I pose, you will find now that you are a bit longer in your stance and that you feel longer and stronger in this pose. Again, stay for three to five breaths.
- Folding from the hips, place your hands on either side of the front foot.
- Step the right leg back to the left leg, feet hip width apart.
- Staying on the balls of the feet—with feet hip width apart—lift the hips high, arriving into Downward Facing Dog pose. (**Note**: if getting to the floor is not for you today, use a chair set in front of you—on

your yoga mat—to prevent the chair from slipping. Do this pose with hands holding the outer edges of the seat of the chair).

6. Adho Mukha Svanasana—Downward Facing Dog

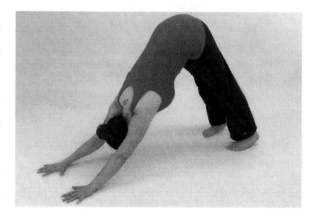

- Push away from the floor with both the hands and the feet.
- Lift the hips high, lengthening both the torso and the legs.
- Though the heels are not on the floor, internally work to reach into the inner heels. This will help draw navel to the spine.
- Four actions keep the shoulders safe in this upper-body weight-bearing pose:

  a. Light outward rotation of the shoulders.

  b. Reaching into the heels of the hands, more on the thumb side. Bear into the base of the index-finger knuckle while all fingertips/thumbs, and base of all the fingers/thumbs also push the floor.

  c. Creating space between the shoulder blades and using your breath to enhance that.

  d. Drawing the head of the humerus (upper arm) slightly deeper into the shoulder joint. Focus on a deeper connection where the upper arm meets the shoulder joint.

7. High Plank

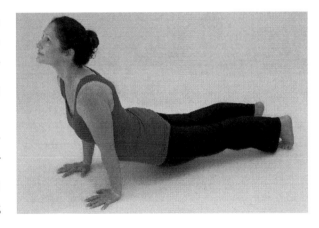

- Keeping the elbows straight, unfold from the hips, coming into a straight line from heels to the shoulders.
- Keep the actions of 1 and 2 above and spread wide both the collarbones and the shoulder blades.
- Still reaching into the inner heels, draw navel to the spine. Stay one or two breaths. Keep your hands and feet as they are, and on an exhale begin to move into the next pose.

8. Urdhva Mukha Svanasana—Upward Facing Dog.

- Drop the hips slightly, inviting a light backbend into the upper rib cage, and begin to lift your gaze.
- To keep from working too hard in your lower back, still reach into the inner heels of the feet, lengthen the tailbone down, and draw the navel to the spine.
- Move the sternum forward and up, or as we say quite often in yoga, "let the heart lead."
- Stay one or two breaths and on an exhale, return to your Downward Facing Dog pose.

9. Adho Mukha Svanasana—Downward Facing Dog

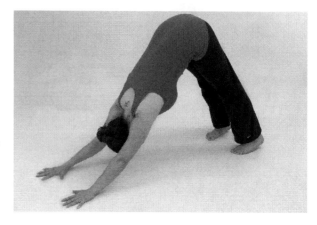

- Whenever you can, come into Downward Facing Dog from Plank or Upward Facing Dog without moving your feet. Your body will learn to tolerate and accommodate the transitions between these three poses as they should all be done from the same hand-to-foot distance. This will happen with consistent practice. If you need to adjust for tight hamstrings, lower-back or calf muscles—or joint issues in the knee, ankle or foot—listen to your body and practice safely.

From this pose, step the left leg to between the hands and repeat the Warrior sequence leading with the left leg.

B. Sun Salute sequence (see Sun Salute from Sequence 1: Morning Sequence), and include sandwiching in one or more of the following poses, depending on time.

1. Parivrtta Parsvakonasana—Revolved Side Angle Pose

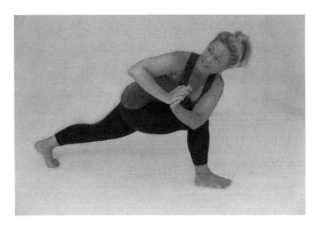

- From the lunge position (after pose A5 or A9 of Sun Salute, Sequence 1 Morning Sequence) while hands are one on either side of the right foot, extend the right arm forward, hand palm down, held higher than the head.
- Turn the head and rib cage to look underneath the armpit behind you, aiming to where the ceiling meets the wall.
- Inhale and reach down and back into the inner back heel and up to the fingertips.
- Open up through the back of the knee.
- Exhale, finding more turn possible through the waistline and rib cage because of how the left hand uses the leverage of pressing into the floor.
- Hold for three to five breaths and return to the lunge, completing that Sun Salute.
- Then, repeat Revolved Side Angle Pose on the other side with the next repetition of the Sun Salute.

2. Chaturangua—Low Plank

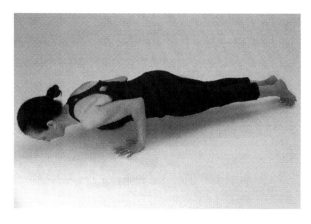

- In the Sun Salute, after arriving into High Plank (pose A6 from Morning Sequence), lower the body weight to Push Up pose, hovering just slightly away from the floor, and hold for a breath or two.
- Here, the elbows are held over the wrists, hands shoulder width apart, and the elbows point back—not out to the side.
- If High Plank is too difficult, rest the shins at the floor, though note that the body is straight from the knees to the shoulders/head.

3. Vasisthasana—T-Stand—from High Plank

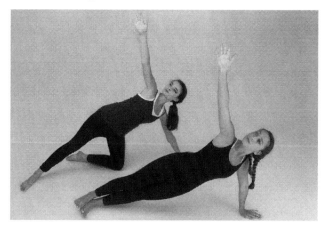

- (Sandwich in after High Plank (pose A6 from Morning Sequence) or after Chaturangua, above.)
- Drop the right knee, keep the left leg straight behind its hip, turn the left leg out resting the sole of the foot on the floor, and lift the left arm straight up (arms/body are like a letter T).
- The lower hand must stay directly under or slightly ahead of the shoulder.
- Stay a few breaths and come to all fours to then extend the right leg straight back behind the right hip.

- Do exactly the same on the other side. This is a beginner's version while the option below is more intermediate/advanced requiring more strength of the shoulder girdle, back and core.
- Keeping both legs straight, pivot off of both feet, lifting the outside arm straight up.
- The top leg rests in front of the bottom leg, edges of the feet with the floor, and the legs are both straight. Another variation is to stack the feet, which requires more strength and agility for the ankles, as well as more strength of the shoulder girdle and core muscles.
- Drop the inside (lower leg) knee to pivot off the back foot.
- Come to all fours and repeat on the other side.

C. Parivrtta Trikonasana—Revolved Triangle

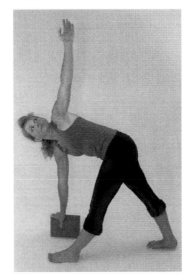

- Step feet wide apart while holding the yoga block in your left hand.
- Turn the right leg out ninety degrees and turn upper body to the right, facing in the direction of the front foot, keeping both legs straight and feet flat at the floor.
- Turn the back foot well forward and do not "walk the tightrope." Thus, walk the right foot slightly to the right. Weight is lightly to the inner edges of the feet.
- Take the right hand behind you, back of the hand to the small of the back, and extend the left arm forward as you exhale and fold forward, from the hips.
- Keep the left arm reaching actively forward as you inhale.
- Exhale, ground the legs and revolve the torso to the right.
- Inhale and get your bearings.
- Exhale and place the left hand/block on the floor where your left foot would have been. As you use the block also for grounding,

notice how the left hip can keep moving forward while giving attention to the counter action of moving the right hip back.

- Inhale, and lift the right arm out to the right and around/up toward the ceiling. Turn t look up to the right hand. If you have a compromised right shoulder, keep the right hand and arm as they are, behind you..

- Let the work of the bottom three limbs help the body revolve any amount more to the right. Maintain extension of the spine.

- Inhale to come out of the pose, in an upward spiral, keeping the legs, arms, and back straight, while noticing how the back body brings you up against gravity. The unfolding in yoga uses the strength of the back and builds it as well.

- Return to starting position and revolve the feet to repeat the pose to the left..

D. Sarvangasana—Shoulder stand or Candle Pose

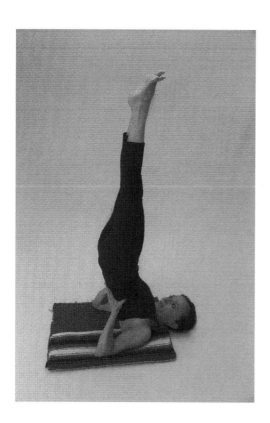 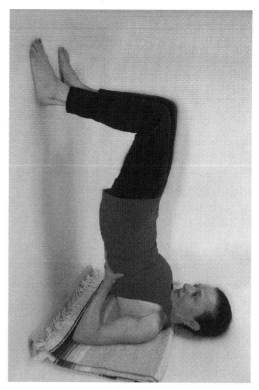

This is considered the "Mother of all Poses," according to B. K. S. Iyengar. It is used as a prescription for improving the health of the thyroid, for lengthening and releasing the back of the neck, for building core strength—especially in the back body—and for conditioning the cardiovascular system. In addition, shoulder stand enhances listening skills.

- Fold two blankets so that they are about two feet by two feet, and place them on the yoga mat. For beginners, set up at the wall and make sure the blankets are somewhat close to the wall so that your feet can walk up the wall and use the wall for support.
- Fold the yoga mat over the blankets to help ensure that the arms do not slip.
- Lie down on your back so that the shoulders and torso are supported by the blanket/yoga mat, and the head is slightly lower on the yoga mat.
- If using the wall, walk the feet up the wall to lift the hips, bringing the knees to ninety degrees.
- Extend the arms below you, and take the time to tuck each shoulder in turn underneath you bit more.
- Keeping the elbows on the floor, bring the hands up—palms against the back—to support the back.
- Take one leg straight up toward the ceiling and if your core strength allows, take both legs straight up.
- Try to keep the elbows close and from sliding out to the side.
- Make sure not to turn the head at any time.
- Build time here, eventually trying to stay for one to five minutes.
- Reach into the big-toe mounds as in Mountain Pose.
- To come out of the pose, return feet to the wall. Drop the hips, roll to the right side, and rest the head in the right arm for thirty seconds to one minute. Try to keep the body even to allow the blood volume to readjust so you will come upright without feeling light headed. Intermediate students will enter and exit shoulder stand using Plough pose to release the extensor muscles of the spine.

E. Traction Twist

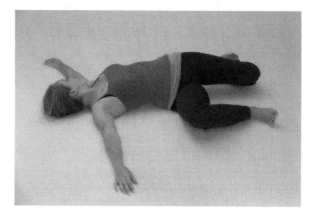

- Resting on your back, make sure to first plant your feet under your knees to get the proximity of the feet. Then, walk the feet to the edges of your mat wider than the hips. Drop the knees to the right, aiming to keep the left thigh with the line of the torso and the left shin perpendicular to the body. Prop with a block under the left knee to accommodate for a tight hip or knee. Draw the lower ribs toward the floor.
- Arms are held out to the side, and the head turns to look opposite the knees. Stay up to one minute and repeat on the other side.
- This pose releases the lower back due to tractioning the psoas, which originates on the inside of the lumbar spine. The psoas is also the deep core muscle that holds the memory of trauma, so this release is a wonderful way to let go of unnecessary stress both physically and emotionally in the body.

F. Peaceful Lake Pose

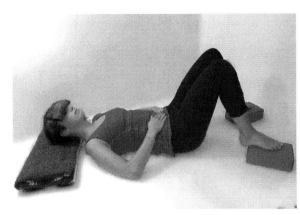

- Draw the knees up and keep the feet wider than the hips, rest the knees against each other at the midline of the body.
- Rest the hands at the soft part of the belly.
- Stay another two-to-five minutes, breathing into the belly, letting the belly rise and fall with each breath.

Strengthening Sequence At-a-Glance

Warrior Sequence:

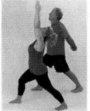 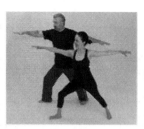 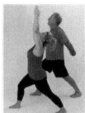 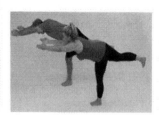 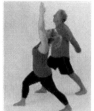

A1. Virabhadrasana I / Warrior I

A2. Virabhadrasana II / Warrior II

A3. Virabhadrasana I / Warrior I

A4. Virabhadrasana III / Warrior III

A5. Virabhadrasana I / Warrior I

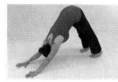 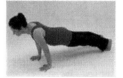 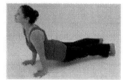 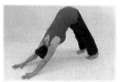

A6. Adho Mukha Svanasana / Downward Facing Dog

A7. High Plank

A8. Urdhva Mukha Svanasana / Upward Facing Dog

A9. Adho Mukha Svanasana / Downward Facing Dog

B. *Sun Salute:*

See sequence photos from Morning Sequence. Insert B1-B3 poses as shown:

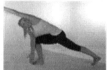 or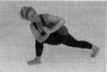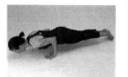

B1. Parivrtta Parsvakon-asana / Revolved Side Angle Pose (after A5 or A9 from Sun Salute)

B2. Chaturangua / Low Plank (after A6 from Sun Salute)

B3. Vasisthasana / T-Stand from High Plank (after A6 from Sun Salute or Chaturangua, left)

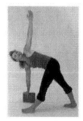 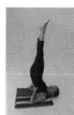 or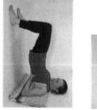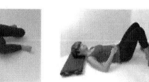

C. Parivrtta Trikonasana / Revolved Triangle

D. Sarvangasana / Shoulder stand or Candle Pose

E. Traction Twist

F. Peaceful Lake Pose

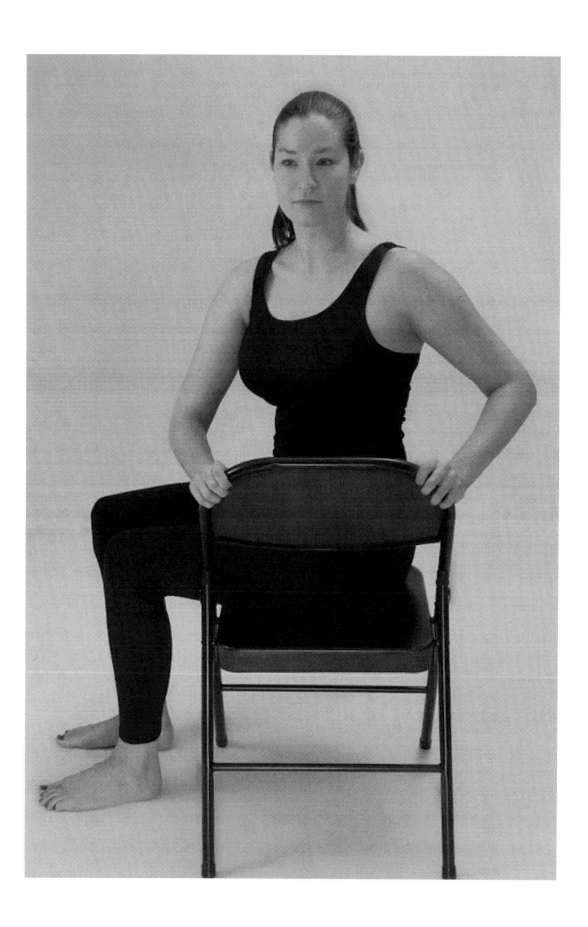

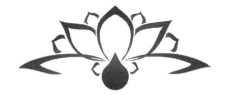

SEQUENCE 3: DETOX SEQUENCE

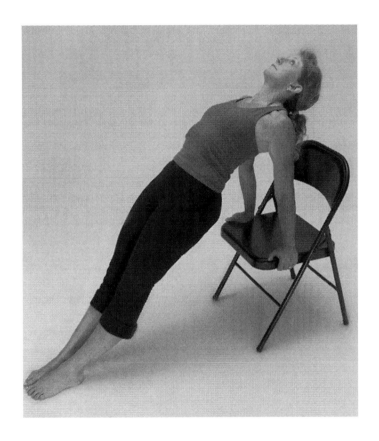

The body is your temple. Keep it pure and clean for the soul to reside in. —B. K. S. Iyengar

Intention of the Detox Sequence

The intention of the detox sequence is to get rid of unnecessary tension, toxins and negativity, thus addressing the mind-body-spirit connection. This yoga sequence is built on the foundation of using twists.

Physiologically, when we twist, depending on the pose chosen and the angles of work against gravity, we can affect the stretch of the smaller muscles that run between each vertebra along with muscles that run diagonally to the ribs nearby and the superficial muscles of the back too. When we unwind from a twist, the smaller muscles especially are willing to stay stretched out to a degree, and we feel more limber in our spine and rib cage. Discs and the nerves that run out into the body from inbtween the vertebrae have more room. We are thus not limited due to tense back muscles and/or impingement. Instead, we can access and accomplish more with our increased freedom of movement. Equally, twisting movement of the body begins to detoxify our organs, too. As we move into a twisting posture, blood is squeezed out of organs and tissues. Once we come out of a twist, the surge of blood coming back in to the blood vessels provides perfusion that has a wonderful detoxifying effect.

Interestingly enough, the mind-body effect of practicing yoga postures translates to a cleansing effect of negative thoughts as well. Negative thoughts build up emotional walls that hamper our thought process. Think of how easy it is to dwell on worry and fear while the entire time this overshadows productive participation and enjoyment of daily life. Negative thoughts are toxic to how we get to grow and evolve as human beings. Here is an opportunity to get rid of what we do not need.

> **Oil to use internally:** 2 drops of lemon in water (use glass or metal container).

> **Oil(s) to apply topically:** 1 drop metabolic blend (dilute in a base of fractionated coconut oil). Apply to stomach around the navel. Rub in a circular clockwise motion.

> **Oils to diffuse:** 4 drops grapefruit.

Lemon is well known for its detoxifying qualities. If you'd like to see how powerful lemon is with synthetic substances/chemicals, try putting a drop of lemon oil on Styrofoam or a balloon that has been blown up. Within seconds you will see lemon oil get to work and start dissolving anything that is not carbon based.

This is powerful if you think about how many toxins we have inside our bodies. We are constantly exposed to harmful chemicals and toxins in the air, from the food we eat, and from our personal care products—to name a few.

Any type of exercise releases toxins that are stored in the body. Without a powerful impetus to get them to leave the body, they simply become reabsorbed and have the potential to create even greater harm.

Using lemon oil in water is delicious, is not acid (and therefore, will not harm your teeth). It's a powerful ally to help break down those toxins and—together with good hydration—flush them out of the body for good.

> **Note**: Please be sure that your lemon oil is approved for internal use.

Metabolic Blend
This blend contains such oils as cinnamon, ginger, lemon, grapefruit, and peppermint. The synergistic benefits of these oils have been shown to help promote healthy metabolism, stimulate the endocrine system, calm the stomach and promote a positive mood. (If you pre-fer these oils in your water, they work nicely to purify and cleanse the body as well.)

Grapefruit is known for its energizing and invigorating effects. It helps reduce mental and physical fatigue, and is renowned for its cleansing and purifying benefits. It is frequently used in weight-loss products to support healthy metabolism.

If you read the description of cilantro in Sequence 2, you will remember that detoxification is a key factor in developing strength. As part of that chain, we must recognize that we won't be able to detoxify if we don't let go of the negative feelings and actions we use to *govern our physical bodies*.

How many times do we stand in front of a mirror and criticize our bodies? Our hips are too big and show cellulose, our chest is too small (or too big), our thighs are too jiggly—these comments add to negative energy we hold onto that doesn't allow us to become who we were meant to become. Your body is your temple, the vessel that carries you through your earthly life to participate fully in the myriad of experiences around you.

Honor your body. Treasure it. Love it. Express gratitude for it. Ask it for forgiveness for any verbal, emotional, and physical abuse you have heaped on it. Connect to it. Promise it that your relationship with it is changing for the better. (It can be very enlightening to write your body parts a letter, then listen to what they say in response). As you breathe in the tangy aroma of grapefruit essential oil, choose to increase your resolve to eradicate harmful habits in the way you treat your physical body. Then, you will be better able to detox without adding more sludge to clear out in the future.

> **Props needed:** Yoga mat, two blocks, one strap, yoga blanket, yoga bolster

> **Practice preparation:** Drink plenty of water, before, during and after this sequence. Practice in a comfortably warm environment. Breathe fully and deeply, as you rid the body of toxins through the breath as well. Deep breathing will help you learn to move slowly and mindfully through transitions between your poses as well as to find ease in the depth of each pose.

Suggested length of time in each pose: Beginning yogis: 20–40 seconds, Advanced Yogis: 40–60 seconds. This sequence is more about flushing and releasing; awareness of your range of motion should be your focus rather than time in each pose. When your body becomes more accustomed to deep twists, you'll notice that you will more comfortably move to a deeper range of movement. You'll find more mobility from having practiced a deeper twist. Remember that as your smaller muscles allow you to twist deeper, you'll cleanse out your organs more thoroughly.

Insights about this sequence: Once we have released negative emotions, anxious feelings, and stress through this detoxification sequence, we should feel open—not vulnerable. We should be ready to both give and to receive, and we might easily arrive at a place where we have clarity. Thus, the alignment of the restorative pose at the end of this sequence will allow us the potential of all of these benefits. Be sure to spend ample time—five to twenty minutes—in the very last pose, which is Supta Baddha Konasana.

Detox Sequence

A. Tadasana—Mountain Pose to Urdhva Hastasana—Volcano

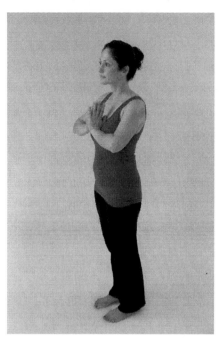 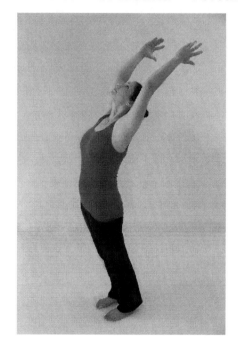

B. Utkatasana—Powerful Pose with a twist

- As you sit deeper into this imaginary chair, from arms reaching overhead, bring hands together in Namaskarasana, turn from the waistline to the right, and hook the left elbow on the outer right knee.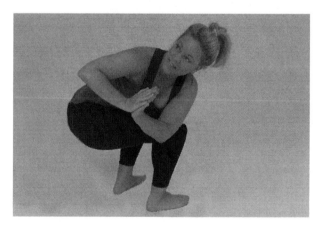
- Inhale, come back to center with the general chair pose alignment.
- Exhale, and turn from the waistline to the left.
- With hands in prayer, hook the right elbow on the outer left knee.

- Inhale, and come back to center, reaching hands overhead.
- Continue the inhalation and return first to Volcano and then back to Mountain pose before doing the other side.

C. Parivrtta Parsvakonasana—Revolved Side Angle Pose

- Lunge the left leg back, bending the right knee to ninety degrees and placing the hands on the floor—one on either side of the front foot.
- Keep the left hand as it is, helping to bear the weight of the body.

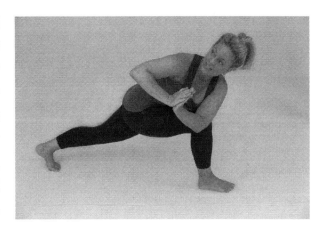

- Take the right hand out to the side—or straight ahead forward, palm down and hand higher than the head—as you begin to revolve the rib cage to the right.
- Look under the armpit to the wall behind you, keeping your gaze up and back.
- The left hand is in charge of this twist, using the floor below for leverage to help the ribcage to turn more to the right. Stay, breathe deeply, and lengthen in the body from the inner back heel to the fingertips, as you twist any amount more.
- Come unwinding out of this twist with an inhalation.
- Placing both hands down, exhale, and step back the right leg into Plank.
- Inhale, and give the body relief while going into Downward Facing Dog.
- Exhale, and step forward the left leg to between the hands to repeat this pose twisting to the left side.

- As you come out of the pose the same way—Plank, to Downward Facing Dog—rest in Child's pose.
- An intermediate form of this pose is to take the elbow to the opposite outer knee and bring the hands into Namaskarasana, aiming to point the top elbow toward the ceiling.

D. Seated Bharadvajasana

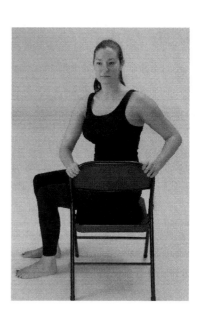

- Sit in a chair turned sideways to the back of the chair.
- Legs should be hip width and feet parallel to each other at the floor.
- If the back of the chair is on your right, exhale, and turn from the waistline to the right, placing the hands at the back of the chair. One hand pushes and the other hand pulls you into the twist.
- Inhale, press down the feet into the floor, draw the navel to the spine, and lift up the ribs off the hips.
- Exhale, and turn any amount more.
- Take the back hand (the right hand here), and place the hand in the seat of the chair—behind the right hip.
- Now the right hand pushes again—this time down into the seat of the chair—and helps you sit up taller, too. Stay another breath or two and inhale to come out of the pose.
- Turn to the other side to repeat the twist.

E. Purvottanasana in the chair

Traditionally, this pose is done from the floor, but is a lot of work on the shoulders, wrists, ankles, and lower back. Here is a kinder way to build the strength of these areas. The lengthening of the torso here, in between the twisting poses of the previous and the next pose will help to aid digestion.

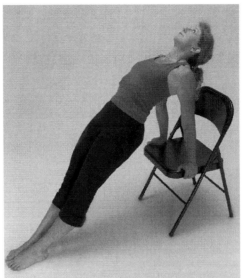

- Sitting centered at the front edge of the chair, place the hands alongside the edges of the seat of the chair behind the hips.
- Walk the feet ahead, and begin to lift the weight of the hips, coming into a reverse plank (facing upward, straight in the body from heels to the head).
- Bring the soles of the feet to the floor—rolling the inner edges of the feet lightly toward the floor—and spread the collarbones and the shoulder blades.
- Inhale, and lift your gaze, being careful not to drop the head back, but finding a neutral alignment for the neck to follow the spine.
- Lengthen the tailbone down, and draw the navel to the spine.
- Inhale as you work with light actions and exhale to come gently out of the pose.

F. Uttanasana in the chair

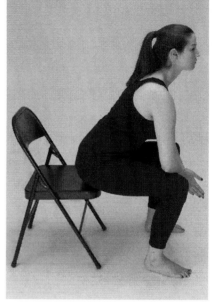

- Stay sitting at the front edge of the chair, and begin to fold from the hips while extending in the spine.
- Place elbows on the thighs and maintaining a straight spine, press down into the floor lightly with the legs, draw the navel more toward the spine, draw the shoulder blades down the back, and actively lengthen the back of the neck upward.
- Stay a couple of breaths, and then go into flexion, rounding the back like in cat pose. Continue to lower the upper body toward the floor, until the head and arms are hanging. If you are tight in your back or hamstrings, and going all the way to the floor is not comfortable, then place a block under your hands.
- Breathe deeply, and walk the arms between the legs to clasp the legs of the chair. Tug lightly with the arms and notice the hip strengthening.
- Inhale, let go, come up slowly and place elbows at the knees again. Take on the same actions as before, while the back is extending again. Stay for a few breaths. This will allow you to come up without feeling light headed.

G. Malasana preparation

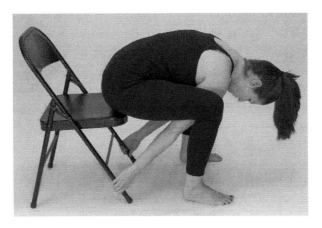

- Roll up a yoga blanket and stand on it— feet a little bit wider than hips, slightly turned out, with the heels on the roll of the blanket and the front of the foot on the floor.
- Begin to squat so that you can drop the weight of your hips while keeping the body mostly upright and the gaze ahead. Advanced students may not need to use the rolled up blanket, as their heels can meet the floor.
- Find the chance to go deep enough to rest elbows against inner knees while hands are in prayer position.
- The elbows and inner legs work lightly against each other.
- Broaden the collarbones and shoulder blades.
- Lengthen the back of the neck upward.
- Ease back to standing using Chair pose, or fold first into Uttanasana, standing forward bend, and ten unfold from the hips, to standing upright.

H. Ardha Matysendrasana—Half Lord of the Fishes

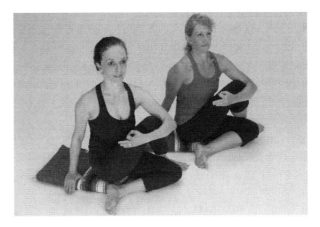

- Sit on a folded blanket with the right leg in front, right knee bent, and the leg turned onto its side while the right heel is close to the pubic bone.

- The left foot is either planted aligned with the left hip or across the midline on the outside of the right knee—left foot flat with the floor.
- At first, hold on to the left knee with both hands, draw yourself upright, and press the legs into the floor, anchoring the left sitting bone especially.
- Turn to the left, hugging the left knee with the right arm or elbow, and place the left hand on the floor behind the left hip so as to prop the body more upright and to sit taller.
- Inhale, reach down with the right leg and left hand, lift the ribs off the hips and exhale, turning any amount more to the left.
- Stay a few breaths and inhale to come out of the pose.
- Switch placement of the legs to do the twist to the right.

I. Apanasana—Knee to the Chest

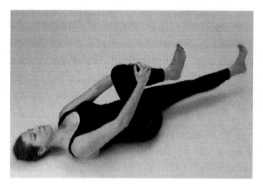 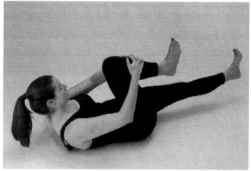

- Resting on your back, bring the right knee to the chest, and hold the shin with both hands—elbows fairly straight.
- The hands pull and the shin resists.
- To engage the core muscles more, lift the head and shoulders.
- Keep the left leg hovering from the floor, and reach into the inner heel of the left leg. This is the primary action of this pose.
- With each inhalation and exhalation, switch legs, making sure to incorporate the isometric work of the arms and shin working against each other as well as trying to lengthen the long leg.
- Do six to twelve sets, hug the knees, and rest.

- If the neck is weak or gets tired, leave the head resting on the floor.
- Try to be absolutely still throughout the transitions and allow only the limbs to move.

J. Jathara Parivartanasana—Revolved Stomach Pose

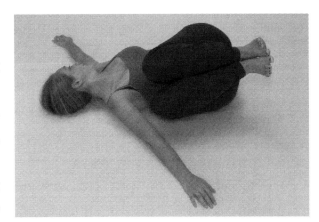

- Lying on your back, bring both knees to the chest, and set the arms wide on the floor—out to the side with palms up.
- Keeping the knees close to the body and feet flexed, exhale, and drop the knees together to the right, aiming to touch the knees to the right elbow, without letting the weight of the legs rest.
- Inhale and bring the legs back to center; exhale, and repeat to the left.
- Do three sets, and then hug the knees.
- When the strength of the arms holds the weight of the legs, the muscles of the lower back relax to recover.

K. Supported Supta Baddha Konasana—Reclined Bound Angle Pose—

- Reclined Bound An-
gle pose is a great
chest, shoulder, and
hip opener—and a
supported backbend
as well.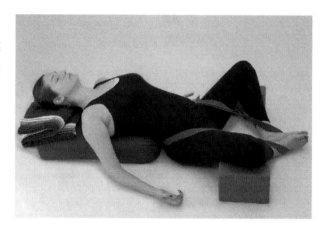
- Place the yoga bol-
ster in the center
of the mat, length-
wise with the mat.
At one end, a folded yoga blanket will serve as an elevation
for the head (like a pillow.
- Sit in front of the bolster with feet together and knees turned
out to each side. Have a yoga block ready beside each knee.
- Next, use the strap to pull and hold the feet together closer to
the body. Pull the end of the strap through the buckle creating
a loop. Wrap the strap from around the hips to include the feet,
and cinch it up. Make sure to have the tail of the strap facing
you, so that you are able to tighten it more as needed. Also, the
strap should be at the sacrum, the center of the pelvis behind
you, not at the waistline.
- Prop one block under each knee. This will support each hip/leg
as well as the lower back from the stress that can occur when
there is not a prop under each knee. As your body opens up to
the support of the blanket, bolster, blocks, and strap, make sure
to rest the arms beside you with palms turned upward to maximize the effect of gravity to open the front of the shoulders.
- Bring your focus to your breath. Savor the sweetness of feeling
"open" while being supported. Together, these two factors allow
you to find and be who you are meant to be in life, unencum-
bered by whatever might hold you back.

- When you are ready to come out of the pose, reach down to release the buckle, straighten your legs and flex your feet. Reach into the inner heels. If the support was adequate, your lower back will be well supported with this alignment as well.
- Relax, and stay here for one-to-five minutes.
- Roll to your right and continue to rest if needed and then sit upright. You will now find yourself refreshed and ready.

Detox Sequence At-a-Glance

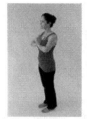 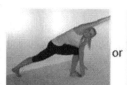 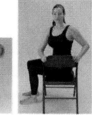 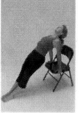

or

| A. Tadasana / Mountain Pose | B. Utkatasana / Chair Pose with a twist | C. Parivrtta Parsvakonasana / Revolved Side Angle Pose | D. Seated Bharadvajasana | E. Purvottananasana in the Chair | F. Uttanasana in the Chair |

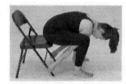 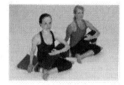 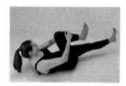 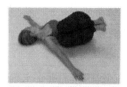 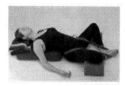

| G. Malasana Preparation | H. Ardha Matysendrasana / Half Lord of the Fishes | I. Apanasana / Head to the Knee | J. Jatharta Parivartanasana | K. Supported Supta Baddha Knasana / Reclined Bound Angle Pose |

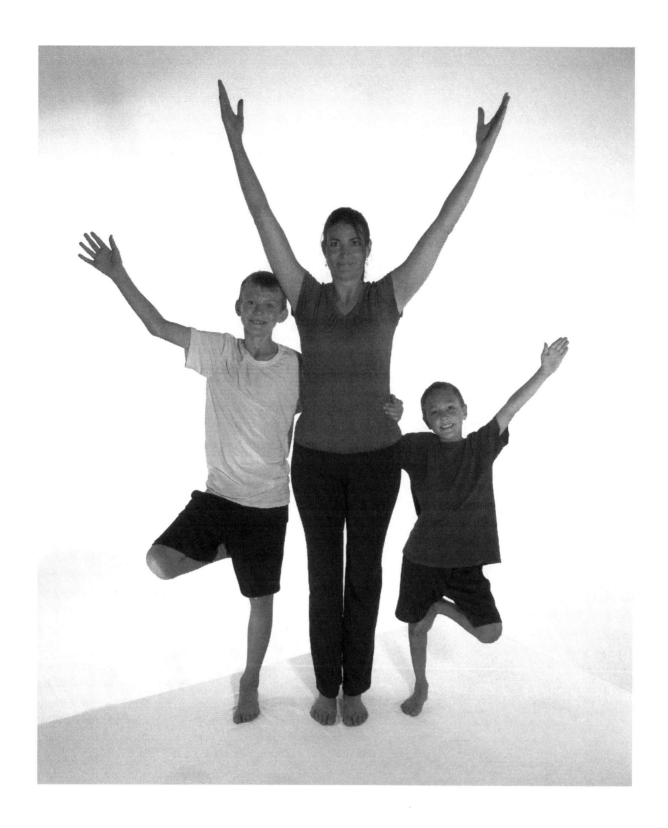

SEQUENCE 4: MOM/DAD AND ME (PARTNER) SEQUENCE

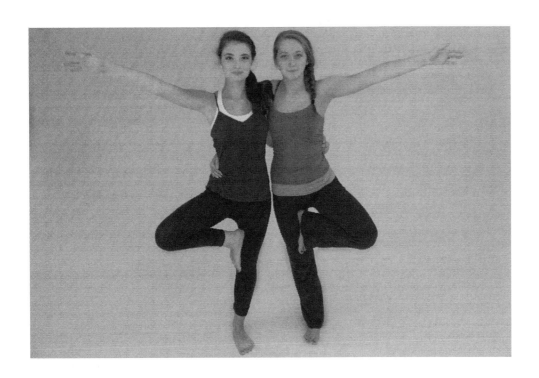

Intention of the Partner Sequence

The intention of this sequence is to bond, nurture relationships, and to recognize that life is better when we live, work, and play together. When we devote time to one another, and make one another the priority, it becomes an opportunity to learn from one another in so many ways. We learn balance and patience, we learn to adjust for one another, support one another, seek out fun, pull one another up, and be more open with one another. We feel accepted and valued when someone else wants to spend time with us, and we realize how valuable it is to do that for others. We learn along the way to appreciate each person's gifts. We give others time to shine. We grow together with memories made from having spent time together, and we evolve as human beings.

    Note: This sequence is ideal for after-school connection.

    Oil(s) to apply topically: One drop of grounding blend on the bottoms of feet and over the heart. One drop of repellent blend on the back of the neck and over the heart.

    Oils to diffuse: Invigorating blend.

Grounding Blend

This blend can include such oils as spruce, ho wood oil, frankincense, blue tansy, and blue chamomile in a base of fractionated coconut oil. There has been much written about the benefits of starting your yoga sequence with a pure and potent grounding blend. (See sequences 1, 4, and 5.) Outside the protective shelter of our homes, the world can be a stressful, confusing place. The pressures of school and social interactions can take their toll on children—no matter what their age.

As was discussed in the first sequence, a good grounding blend can evoke feelings of tranquility and balance. Using a grounding blend during the first few minutes after school or just before bed can help parents and children bond as they work to enhance communication and create long-lasting relationships.

Repellent Blend

This blend Includes such oils such as lemon, eucalyptus, citronella, and other oils that protect against insects and other predators. The fresh, light citrus scent resulting from this oil blend is wonderfully invigorating. There is a metaphor to be used as we consider the effectiveness of the repellent blend in helping to manage exposure to biting insects: we can intentionally create a connection in our minds between physical "biting predators" (in this case, insects) and energetic biting predators. In this way, we can allow the repellent blend to support us in keeping our "energetic" protective shield high, which has several benefits. First, it helps us feel safe and in control of our own lives despite what is thrown at us from the outside. If we were feeling vulnerable already, it helps restore our sense of trust in our strength and also helps us access strength from our Higher Power and loved ones.

Focus on the locations suggested for topical application—the back of the neck, where we typically carry stress and heaviness, and the heart, which is the organ that represents both our vulnerability and ability to connect with others.

The other powerful benefit resulting from the connection we draw between physical and energetic biting predators is that we can use the aroma of the repellent blend as a reminder to create and maintain healthy relationship boundaries. Each of us—either due to genetics, environmental exposure, or both—interacts with our families in a certain way. Add that tendency to real-life stressors, and it's easy for us to disregard healthy boundaries. Either we get too close—where we take too much responsibility for one another—or we insert too much distance because we don't want to feel vulnerable. We don't trust.

We can allow the repellent blend to remind us to interact in healthy ways that connect us in all the ways that matter. We are better able to share how we feel, voice what is important to us, respect someone else's space, listen—and most importantly—keep our hearts open to interpersonal connection, which is how we thrive best.

Because this sequence is all about healthy interdependent interaction, we have two tools at our disposal as we reprogram past genetic patterns and current communication patterns. Use your body to connect while holding your own space. Use repellent blend to remind you how strong you are when you learn to balance a healthy boundary with those you love.

Invigorating Blend

This blend includes such oils as wild orange, lemon, grapefruit, mandarin, bergamot, tangerine, clementine, and vanilla bean extract. An invigorating blend merges the benefits of citrus essential oils to form a unique and harmonious blend. It helps elevate mood, reduce stress, and has natural, potent compounds with cleansing properties.

The mood-elevating properties of the invigorating blend serve as the perfect aromatic "backdrop" to create memories with our children/loved ones. It is likely that your limbic system—as it stores the memory of your partner yoga sequence together with the citrus blend aroma—will recall sweet emotions every time you smell a citrus fruit/oil in the future.

Sequence Instructions:

Live with intention. Walk to the edge. Listen hard. Practice wellness. Play with abandon. Laugh. Choose with no regret. Appreciate your friends. Continue to learn. Do what you love. Live as if this is all there is.
—Mary Radmacher

Props needed: Yoga mat, one-to-two blocks (optional for height difference), one yoga blanket for each partner, one chair per two people.

Practice preparation: Parents—anticipate the practice session and the conversation you want to have with your child/children. Think of encouragement that you want to interject when the time is right. Use words that are age appropriate and consider planning a mantra or meditation for the ending, restorative pose. Your child will learn to anticipate what you have prepared. While this is not absolutely necessary, another approach is to be open to creative play—especially with smaller children—and see what unfolds. No matter what, you will be pleasantly surprised at the outcome, especially if your yoga practice becomes regular.

Suggested length of time in each pose: Considering the element of creative fun, try to stay in each pose about one minute. Enjoy your partner.

Insights about this sequence: Partner poses in yoga have many benefits. They are designed to create a bonding effect between the partners involved and promote both nurturing and trust. They also allow leverage and tractioning from different angles. Physical work against gravity changes, and the support of the partner can take away some of the need for control in balance. This, in turn, allows muscle fibers to work and gain strength from a longer position. Partner poses incorporate an element of fun and help with inviting others to change perspective. This lesson can travel well "off the mat" and lend itself to adjusting to daily hurdles.

Remind yourself to be playful.
—Alexandra Stoddard

In this sequence, sometimes a difference in height may not make a difference. Options will be provided for partners with height differences.

Partner Pose Sequence

A. Tadasana—Mountain Pose

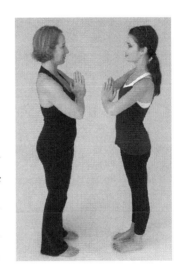

- Stand facing your partner, hands in prayer (Namaskarasana), acknowledging each other while centering in your space. This hand position is a sign of respect and can translate to mean "the honor in me respects the honor in you, that we are here to work together in harmony."

B. Virabhadrasana I—Warrior I

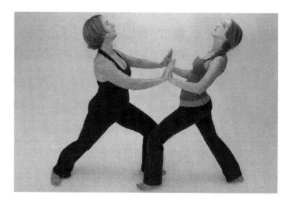

- Stand facing your partner and place both palms against each other shoulder height and shoulder width. When partners are of different heights, then the height of the hands should be halfway between the taller/shorter shoulders.
- Step your right leg forward, knee bent, and your left leg back, leg straight.
- As you press hands into each other, bring the left hip more forward and notice how the calf muscles are deepening their stretch as a result of the hands pushing.
- Lift the rib cage, and notice the small back bend in the upper rib cage. Teaching a backbend to the upper rib cage is the work of Warrior I, so breathe deeply and stand taller together. Do both sides.

C. Virahabhadrasana II—Warrior II

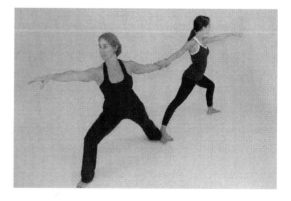

- Turn sideways from each other, rest the outer edges of the feet against each other—this is the "inside leg" and is straight.
- Step the outside leg well away, turn the foot out, and try to come to a ninety-degree bent knee. You are both all on one plane.

- Hold each other from the wrists of the inside (back) hand and turn away to look over the front arm. Your light tug and lean will help you grow your wingspan, invite space into tired shoulders, release tension in the neck, and open the hips.
- Ease back in and turn around to do the other side.

D. Vrksasana—Tree

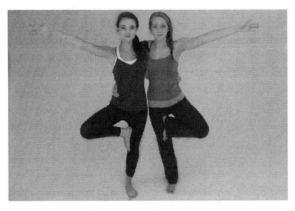 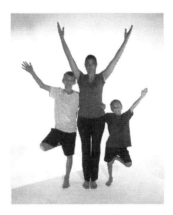

- Stand side by side. Hug your partner at his/her waistline—each person with their inside arm.
- Your inside legs will stay grounded and straight, and your outside legs will prop up at the floor with bent knee turned out or against the inside legs.
- The outside arms will "grow the branches "of the tree. As you reach up, notice that you can stand taller than you might have been able to on your own and that you are able to stay stable longer while together in this pose.

E. Utkatasana—Powerful or Chair Pose (variations) This pose works better when partners are about the same height/weight

1. Simple.

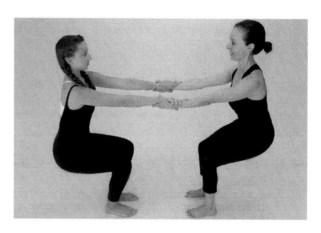

- Stand facing each other; hold each other at the wrists, arms parallel to one another.
- Lean away from each other, keeping Plank in the body. (Plank means, maintaining a straight line between the crown of the head and the ankles). Your sense of balance will help with how close to place your feet away from the feet of your partner.
- Once you both balance how you are leaning away from each other, you can begin to spread the collarbones, root more into the legs, lengthen the front spine, and invite a small backbend into the upper rib cage. Stay here for a few breaths and enjoy the opening of the front body.
- Then, begin to sit back, aiming your sitting bones toward the wall behind you. You will need to lean well away from your partner to balance in this pose and avoid stress in the knees.
- To return, pull toward each other simultaneously, using the strength of your arms/biceps, and come to standing.

2. With a twist

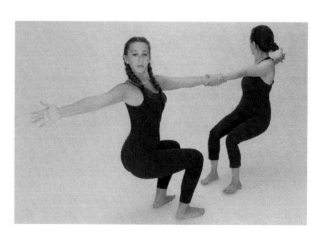

- Holding on to your partner now changes—right wrists are held together and left wrists are held together. Again, your sense of balance will help you with foot placement and the proximity to each other.

- As you sit back to an imaginary chair as in the position above, find your balance point, let go the right arm/hands from each other, turn away from each other to the right. Each person should look at his or her own right hand back behind himself or herself.
- Return together and reclasp the hands holding at the wrists.
- Do the same, letting go and twisting to the left.
- To return, pull toward each other to stand up and to come together as above.

F. Upavista Konasana—Wide-legged Upright Cone

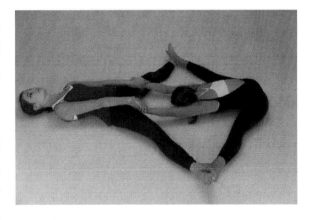

- Sit on the floor, facing your partner. Legs are wide and feet rest against each other.
- Depending on hamstring and lower-back flexibility, you may either catch each other at the hands, wrists, or hold on to a yoga strap between you.
- Begin with one person folding forward, the other leaning back and switch, so that you begin to find a comfortable fold.
- Then, with hands still in the same position, create more of a circular pattern, and make sure to try circling in both directions.

G. Navasana—Boat Pose

This pose works best with people of the similar size but can be improvised with the shorter person putting their feet lower on the legs of their partner. For example, the shorter person would place their feet on the back of the calves of the taller person.

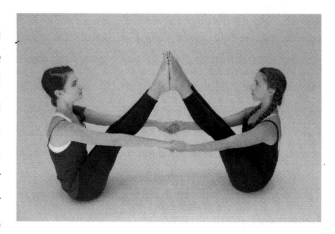

- Sit facing each other and firmly hold each other by the hand or wrist.
- Slowly, place one foot against the foot of your partner—directly across from you—and extend that foot/leg upward until the legs are straight.
- Holding that position, try to do the same with the other foot/leg.
- If your core strength will not allow you to sit in this V position with both of your feet against both of your partners' feet, practice just one side and then the other. Over time, you will be able to do it.
- Try not to round in your back; sit tall by tugging at your partner, and try staying at the top of your sitting bones, reaching out through the crown of the head, while spreading your collar bones.

H. Jathara Parivartanasana—Revolved Stomach Pose.

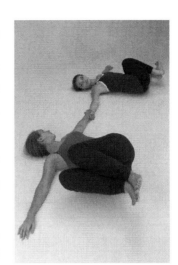

- Lying on the floor, side by side, at arms' length between you and your partner, hold on to a small loop of a yoga strap between you and your partner, or hold your partner by the wrist.
- The free arm reaches out to the side so that the arms create a "T" pattern with the body.
- Draw the knees toward the chest and, with an inhalation, drop the knees away from each other.
- Exhale, and draw back the knees toward the starting position.
- Do four-to-six repetitions—slowly and controlled. This is an incredible strengthening twist and targets the oblique and latissimus dorsi muscles, thus strengthening the lumbar spine, and core muscles in general.
- Turn to lie in the other direction, holding the small loop of the yoga strap or your partner's wrist with the other hands, to do the other side.

I. Adho Mukha Svanansana—Downward Facing Dog

There are many partner variations for Downward Facing Dog, and as you become familiar with your own Downward Facing Dog pose, you will be more resilient in this classic strengthening of the body. Practice doing this pose separate from each other for a few weeks, and learn to build time (try to stay a minute)

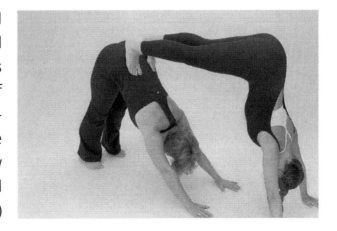

as you build your own inner strength. In the long run, this is a resting pose and used as a transitional pose in-between standing poses and poses from the floor.

- One person does Downward Facing Dog.
- The other partner their hands 8-to-12 inches in front of the partner already in Downward Facing Dog pose, and gently—one foot at a time—places his or her feet on the sacrum/pelvis of that partner. The second person will be practicing a handstand preparation and will be with their body more at a ninety-degree angle, folding from the hips. This is an empowering place for both partners—each in a separate way. The Downward Facing Dog partner will experience a wonderful grounding effect and will have less work in the shoulders. The partner's feet on his or her sacrum will help to ground the heels closer to the floor and take some weight off the shoulders. The person on the bottom will feel as if he or she could stay here a bit longer than anticipated.
- To come out of the pose, the handstand partner on top will again, gently—one leg at a time—step down, and the Downward Facing Dog partner can then come out of the pose. Switch places and then, if needed, rest in Child's pose, separate from each other.

J. Sukhasana—Happy Pose—Twist
1. Facing each other

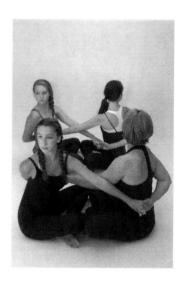

- Sitting on a folded blanket, cross the legs, and sit close enough that your knees are touching.
- Each person takes his or her right hand/arm behind and across their back reaches with their left arm across the midline at a diagonal and beginning to

twist to the right, catches their partner's hand at their partner's back body.

- Legs bear lightly into the floor, and knees bear lightly into the partner's knees.
- Tug with the arms, sit tall, and turn away from your partner.
- Breathe deeply and enjoy staying for a few breaths.

2. Back to back

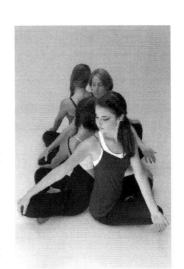

- Sitting on a folded blanket, cross the legs, and sit close enough that you are leaning slightly against the partner behind you.
- Each person reaches their right hand and sets it against their own outer left knee, takes their left hand and catches their partner's right knee back behind them.
- Lean well against each other and twist gently to the left.
- Stay for a few deep breaths, and repeat to the other side.

K. Sukhasana—Happy Pose with Supported Rest

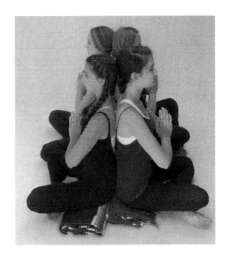

- Sit back to back—each person sitting against the other—on a folded blanket with legs crossed. Another option is to put a rolled up blanket or yoga blocks under each knee to support tight hips.
- Hold Namaskarasana—hands at the heart—and honor the partner behind you, supporting you.

L. Legs in the Chair This is the perfect way to relax the lower back and revive tired legs.

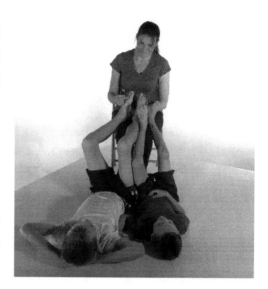

- As you rest on your back with hips and knees (each at ninety degrees), the calves rest in the seat of the chair.
- This is the perfect opportunity to put essential oils on the bottoms of the feet.
- Stay five to twenty minutes, breathe deeply, and enjoy some conversation with your partner while your body is revived with this restorative pose.

Partner Sequence at-a-Glance

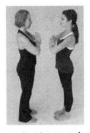 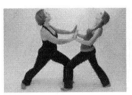 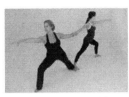 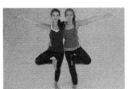 or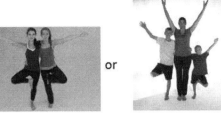

A. Tadasana / Mountain Pose

B. Virabhadrasana I / Warrior I

C. Virabhadrasana II / Warrior II

D. Vrksasana / Tree

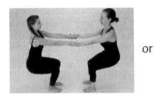 or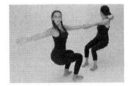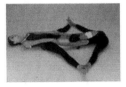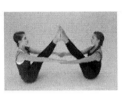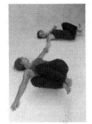

E1. Utkatasana / Simple Chair Pose

E2. Utkatasana / Chair Pose with a Twist

F. Upavista Konasana / Wide Legged Upright Cone

G. Navasana / Boat Pose

H. Jathara Parivartanasana / Revolved Stomach Pose

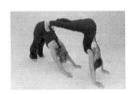 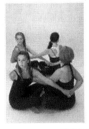 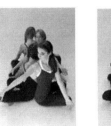 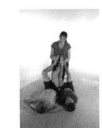

I. Adho Mukha Svanansana / Down Dog

J. Sukhasana / Happy Pose with a Twist — J1. Facing Each Other - J2. Back to Back

K. Sukhasana / Happy Pose with Supported Rest

L. Vipariti Karani / Legs in the Chair

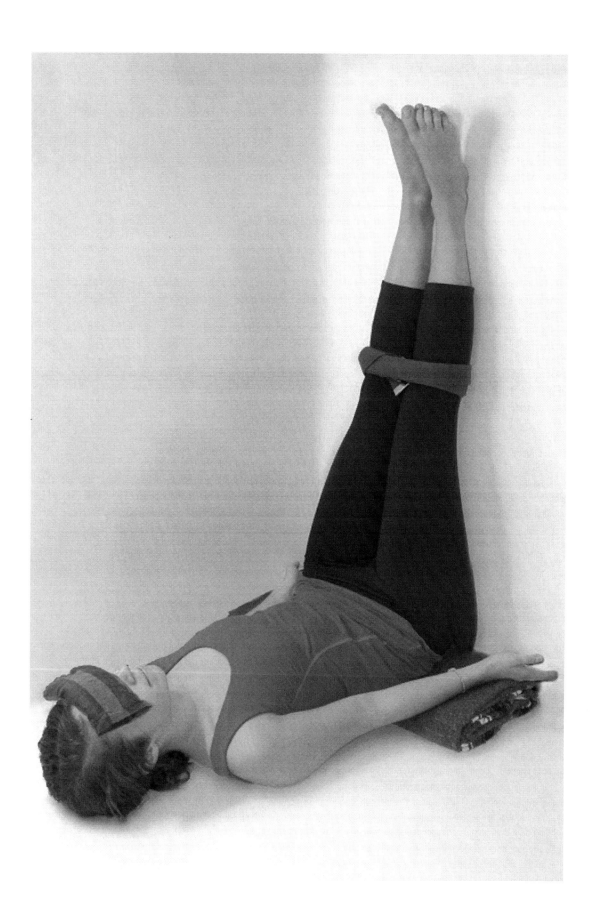

SEQUENCE 5: SLEEP EASY SEQUENCE

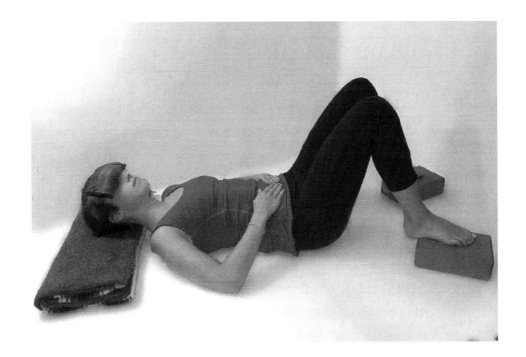

Undisturbed calmness of mind is attained by cultivating friendliness toward the happy, compassion for the unhappy, delight in the virtuous, and indifference toward the wicked.
—The yoga sutras of Patanjali

Intention of the Sleep Easy Sequence

The intention of this sequence is to help the body work off energy from agitation, overstimulation, and apprehension. Such emotions keep the nervous system revved up. At the end of the sequence, the shift is to poses that support the physical structure of the body and thus allow the mind to begin to quiet. Breathing exercises in yoga are categorized as Pranayama practice and are useful here to calm the *monkey mind*— the racing of the mind from one thought to another. The mind quiets and a deeper rest and sleep are accessed. The aim is to then awaken refreshed and revived.

Oil(s) to apply topically: Grounding blend and calming blend—1 drop each on the bottom of each foot, the back of the neck, and over the heart. When applying topically, rub in for approximately 5–10 seconds in a circular, clockwise motion. When finished, rub together palms, cup the nose, and inhale.

Oils to diffuse: 2 drops of respiratory blend and two drops lime.

Grounding Blend

This blend includes oils such as spruce, ho wood oil, frankincense, blue tansy, and blue chamomile in a base of fractionated coconut oil. It promotes tranquility and a sense of balance. Spruce was used by Native Americans for medicinal and spiritual reasons and is still used today to bring harmony to the mind and body. Ho wood, blue tansy, and blue chamomile can soothe sore muscles and joints, promote circulation, and relax the body, while frankincense supports cellular health and overall well-being.

Calming Blend

As mentioned in sequence 2—Strengthening Sequence—this blend includes such oils as lavender, sweet marjoram, Roman chamomile, ylang ylang, sandalwood, and vanilla absolute bean extract. The oils in this blend work together to lessen feelings of tension, calm emotions, and leave a peaceful feeling. It is a wonderful blend to diffuse at bedtime for a restful night's sleep, to calm a restless baby or child, or to help reduce the worry and stress so many of us feel.

When a powerful grounding blend is layered topically *and* used aromatically together with a good calming blend, the relaxing and soothing effects are synergistic. The oils in these blends work together to calm emotions and promote the relaxation and a restful environment that so many of us crave in the evening.

In our society, our minds tend to be overstimulated with visual input—text and writing, electronics, and our own internal agendas of what we think we must accomplish during a given period of time. Our bodies, on the other hand, tend to be more sedentary than they were designed—simply because of the advanced direction of our culture and the professions that are available to us. The result is that we open ourselves to be bombarded by images, ideas, reactions, and brainstorms that leave our brains highly stimulated. Difficulty sleeping has become almost epidemic as we struggle to shut off the constant flow of stimuli and help our brains and bodies become prepared for rest.

When we are tired—or even exhausted—but cannot train our minds and bodies to be "sleepy," we don't get good rest. When we don't get good rest, our bodies are unable to repair themselves during their optimal rebuilding and healing time, and we wake up feeling even more depleted than we did the day before rather than feeling refreshed, strengthened, and ready to create.

Applying these oils topically on the feet gets the oils into the circulatory system very quickly. Targeting the heart and back of the neck helps us remember to slow down and be still, which helps to quiet the mind.

Respiratory Blend

This blend includes such oils as laurel leaf, peppermint, eucalyptus, melaleuca (tea tree), lemon peel, ravensara, and cardamom seed oil. The oils in a respiratory blend work together to help us breathe easier. They soothe the airways and promote clear breathing. When applied topically or diffused at nighttime, this blend calms the senses and promotes sleep.

Most of us are shallow breathers. Think about the last time you focused on breathing so deeply through your nose that you could feel the breath go past your waist. Try it now: it doesn't feel normal, does it?

Breathing deeply is important to a healthy body, mind, and heart. It should also be symbolic of our willingness to experience life beyond a superficial level. Physiologically, it expands our oxygen intake and helps our cells to receive what they need. Emotionally, it helps us get "un-stuck," so that we can become more clear. We can move past fears and grief, and expand our capacity to love ourselves, others, and then receive the love we crave.

Many life and personal success coaches teach that whatever you do just before bed is what you are programming your subconscious to focus on. If you eat junk food and watch violent TV programs, you are setting up your subconscious to be focused on horror and lack. If you use pure essential oils coupled with your own positive intention and/ or affirmations, and take your body through a series of poses meant to show your mind and body support and love, you are giving your subconscious permission to create and heal on your behalf all night long.

Lime is an oil with a beautiful, zesty, fragrant aroma that helps to uplift mood, and balance the mind and body. When diffused, lime oil can help purify the air and promote emotional balance and well-being with its refreshing properties.

As you breathe in the beautiful scent of lime essential oil, take the opportunity to clear any shadows that have been created in your mind or heart during the day. Be open to this truth: What other people say and do define *them*, not you. Choose to be open to the truth that you have an infinite, priceless value—that you have gifts, talents, and characteristics to offer in a way that is specific and unique to *you*. You are the only *you* the world will ever know. Embrace your emotional side. Utilize these quiet moments before your Sleep Easy sequence to reaffirm your commitment to the important emotional connections with the significant people in your life. Get out of your head and into your heart. Enjoy a wonderfully satisfying rest full of sweet dreams.

Sequence Instructions:

Mother nature has the power to please, to comfort, to calm, and to nurture one's soul.
—Anthony Douglas

> **Props needed:** Yoga mat, two blocks, one strap, Yoga blanket, eye pillow

> **Practice preparation**: After you have either applied your oil(s) topically and/or aromatically, and after you have removed all electronic stimuli from around you, make sure your sleeping space is warm and quiet. Make the setup process almost a ritual so that you savor the quieting of the body and mind as you prepare for your practice.

> **Suggested length of time in each pose**: See poses below for specific instructions.

> **Insights about this sequence**: If you are overly tired and cannot get your mind to quiet, omit A—the Moon Salute, and go from B to E. The Moon Salute is designed to allow you to release physical stress and nervous energy. The rest of the sequence will still work well to allow the body to wind down.

The more regularly and the more deeply you meditate, the sooner you will find yourself acting always from a center of peace.
—Donald Walters

Sleep Easy Sequence

In the Moon Salute sequence, spend one breath in each pose. In all other poses in this sequence stay up to one minute depending on your stamina.

Moon Salute. This sequence is designed to allow the release of nervous energy and built-up anxious feelings. It is also an aid to quiet the body.

Though it has some similarities to a Sun Salute, Moon Salute uses Warrior I as the transition to and from the floor. Also, like Warrior I, the first repetition is with the right leg leading, and the second repetition is with the left leg leading. Please see descriptions of poses in the Sun Salute in the Morning Sequence and the description of Warrior I in the strengthening sequence.

1. **Tadasana—Mountain Pose**

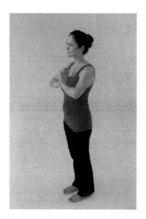

2. **Virabhadrasana I—Warrior I—Right Leg Forward**

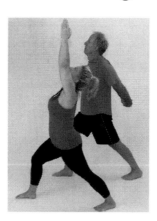

3. **Lunge—Right Leg Forward**

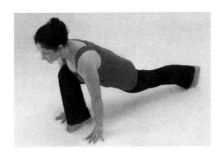

4. **Plank**

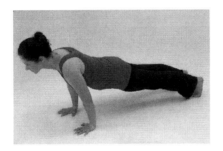

5. **Upward Facing Dog**

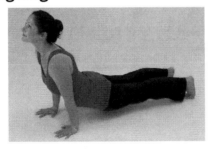

6. **Downward Facing Dog**

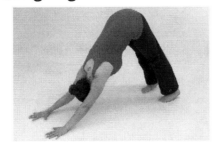

7. Lunge—Right Leg Forward

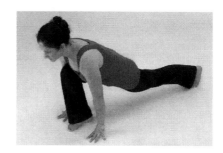

8. Warrior I—Right Leg Forward

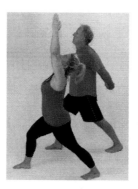

9. Urdhva Hastasana—Volcano

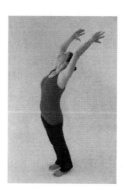

10. **Tadasana—Mountain Pose with Hands in Namaskarasana**

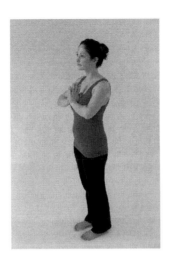

11. Repeat and use left leg in the forward position in poses 2, 3, 7, and 8.

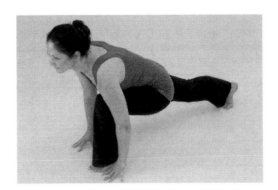

A. Half Uttanasana—Half Standing Forward Fold with Hands at Wall

Forward folds begin to quiet the central nervous system, especially when the head is resting.   Contraindications include degenerative eye issues; if you have retina issues, you know already not to lean forward and put pressure on eyes. Typically, this is safe for pregnant women or people with tight muscles of the back, and legs.

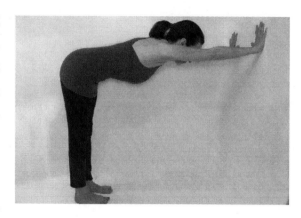

- In this pose, once you fold halfway from the hips so the body is parallel to the floor, the lower back and hamstring muscles begin to stretch, and tension begins to leave the lower back. To maintain safety in forward folds whether are you are very flexible or if you have tight hamstrings or lower-back muscles, "micro-bend" lightly from the knees. The primary action in forward fold is extension of the front of the spine, and that lends to the safety here as well.
- Reach down through the inner heels and up through the sitting bones.
- Start with legs hip-width apart and parallel to each other to disperse the weight of the body equally.
- Fold from the hips.
- Experiment with bending one knee a bit more so the straighter leg can take on the stretch all the way up into the hip joint. Then, switch sides.
- Unfold in the reverse from the hips with a straight back—this will strengthen the extensors of the spine. To come up in a very gentle way, keep a micro-bend in the knees.
- Once you stand upright, roll back the shoulders. As the chest is open, take a slow, deep breath.

B. Balasana—Child's Pose Variations

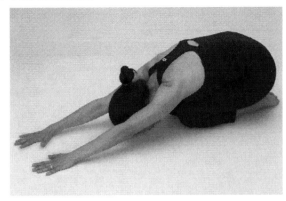

- Stay a minute or longer depending on comfort (another forward fold, in order to quiet central nervous system.) Child's pose is the body's self-preservation pose in times of fear, stress, exhaustion, and vulnerability—both emotionally and physically. This fetal position is how we came into the world and thus is a very soothing pose. It involves flexion of the spine and releases/relaxes the front of the brain.

- In addition, this pose is safe especially for pregnant women. Extra blankets/bolsters may be needed to support the frame of the mother.

- Arms are ahead—with or without a medium-height block under the elbows.

- Arms are behind with palms up toward the ceiling.

- With tall blocks under the hands at arm's reach, the head/neck are held in a neutral position.

- With a twist, place the right hand straight ahead at the floor. The left hand reaches under it with the palm up as the torso and rib cage twist to the right. Rest the head on the floor or on a block, and turn the head to the right to look to the reach of the left hand.

D. Viparita Karani—Legs up the Wall Pose. See Restorative Poses for a description. Stay from 5–20 minutes. This pose relieves tired, aching legs and lower-back discomfort. It is not for pregnant women after twenty weeks.

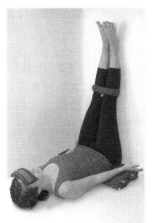

E. Traction Twist

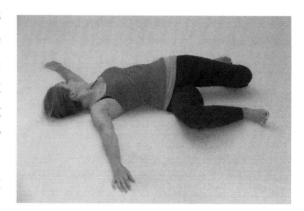

- Stay from 1–5 minutes on each side—this pose will release tension held in the lower back and is not for pregnant women after twenty weeks
- Lying on your back with knees bent and feet planted at the outer edge of the mat, rock the legs to the right, and turn the head to the left. The alignment and weight of the legs will traction the lower back through the psoas muscles, which originate on the inside of the lumbar vertebrae.
- If a tight hip or knee limits you in this pose, place a block under the knee to help hold the weight of the leg without imposing on the joint structure of the knee or hip.

G. Peaceful Lake—Lie on Your Back.

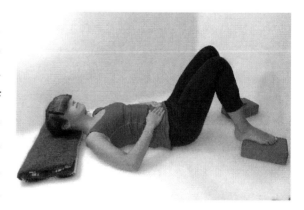

- Stay from 5–10 minutes. This pose is designed to give two advantages— taking excess load off all major joint structures and quieting the front of the brain that is always racing with worry or thinking about a to-do list. Peaceful Lake also helps to focus your breath. Pregnant women should recline with a bolster held up by blocks so that the torso is not below a forty-five-degree angle to the floor.

- Have a yoga blanket or heavy towel folded, and place it under the head so that the head has a slight elevation.
- Place feet under knees—wider than the hips—each foot on a block, with knees resting against each other at the midline of the body.
- Place arms thirty degrees away from the body, and bend in the elbows to bring hands to rest with the fingertips and thumbs resting on the soft part of the belly—not at the lower ribs or hipbones. The belly is the lake. The fingertips are the boats. The people in the boats want the serenity of the movement of the water. Inhale and relax the belly as if the breath could fill the abdomen.
- Exhale, and drop the belly to create the lulling movement of the lake. This is diaphragmatic breathing and strengthens the relationship between the diaphragm and the abdominals. It builds lung capacity and quiets the nervous system.

Sleep Easy Sequence at-a-Glance

A. Moon Salute

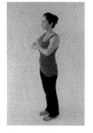
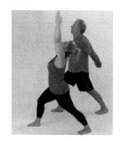
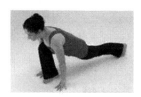
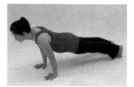

A1. Tadasana / Mountain Pose

A2. Virabhadrasana I / Warrior I

A3. Lunge Right Leg Forward

A4. Plank

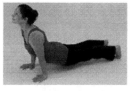
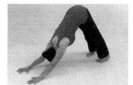
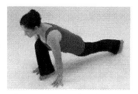
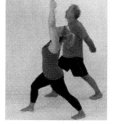
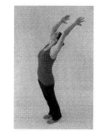

A5. Urdhva Mukha Svanasana / Upward Facing Dog

A6. Adho Mukha Svanasana / Downward Facing Dog

A7. Lunge Right Leg Forward

A8. Virabhadrasana I / Warrior I

A9. Urdhva Hastasana / Volcano Pose

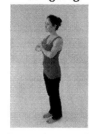
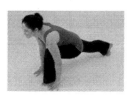
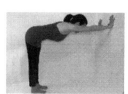
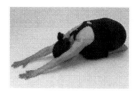
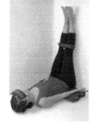

A10. Tadasana / Mountain Pose

A11. Repeat sequence to this point, left leg leading in poses 2, 3, 7 & 8

B. Uttanasana / ½ Standing Fold, with Hands at Wall

C. Balasana / Child's Pose

D. Viparita Karani / Legs up the Wall Pose

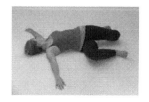
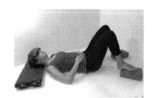

E. Traction Twist

F. Peaceful Lake

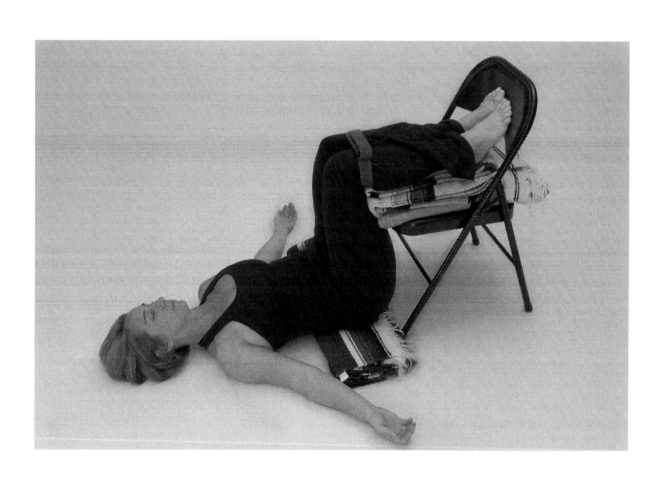

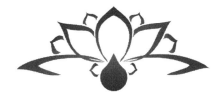

SEQUENCE 6: RESTORATIVE POSES

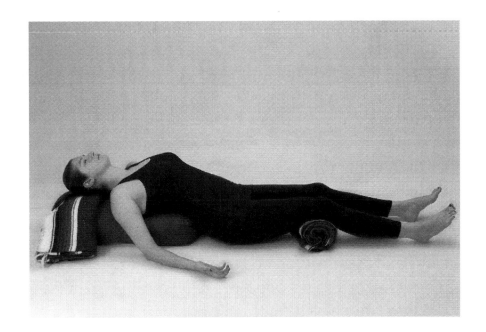

There is no key to happiness—the door is always open. — Mother Teresa

Intention of Restorative Poses

The intention of restorative poses is to save the body's energy by supporting the physical body and allowing muscles to rest deeply. Living in an overly connected world, we are so spent mentally every day that the effect becomes physical lethargy. Furthermore, lack of physical stamina takes a toll on the body's ability to function normally on a cellular level.

Restorative poses in yoga require props to support the framework and thus the joint and muscle structure. These poses allow muscles to let go of their grip and therefore, the energy can be used for other things.

For example, people with compromised bodies can use restorative poses to help with the healing process as the energy reserve can truly be used this way.

Everyone can use restorative poses to help with both physical and emotional realignment with true nature and bring back balance to the body, mind, and spirit. These poses require an investment of time to learn about one's self—not just how we are each unique in our anatomy and thus with the propping that coincides. When we carve out fifteen to twenty or even thirty minutes to spend in each pose and incorporate some deep breathing and meditation, we gain clarity as the mind quiets. An opportunity to move through the daily fog in our lives arrives.

> **Oil(s) to apply topically:** One drop grounding blend on each foot and over the heart (rub in a clockwise circular motion). Female should use one drop of monthly blend on the bottom of each foot and rub it in. Males should dilute and use one drop of thyme on the bottom of each foot. Once the oils are applied, rub together your hands, cup the nose, and inhale deeply.

> **Oils to diffuse:** One drop of clove and two drops of white fir.

Grounding Blend
Much has been said about a good grounding blend. (See Sections 1 and 4 to review.) A good grounding blend is highly complementary to a restorative yoga sequence because the goal is to restore balance, help your muscles to rest deeply, and to replenish and fill. It is much easier to accomplish these goals when you are experiencing tranquility and a sense of balance and when your mind and body are in harmony. Monthly Blend
This blend includes such oils as clary sage, lavender, bergamot, Roman chamomile, cedarwood, ylang ylang, geranium, fennel, carrot seed, palmarosa guatemala, and vitex. Physically, the oils in this blend are

ones that have been traditionally used to balance hormones and manage symptoms of PMS and the transitional phases of menopause. This blend, then, is a powerful ally to supporting a healthy endocrine system and helps to provide temporary respite from emotional swings.

When we think about how a woman can best create, it is when she is true to her nature—when she is immersed in feminine energy. Feminine energy attracts and gathers life—it is warm and it's the very center of creation and flow. A pure monthly blend is a subtle yet powerful way to invite a deep rest and restoration that allows the body, heart, and soul to breathe a collective sigh of contentment.

Thyme is an interesting yet powerful choice for men as they seek to restore balance and fulfillment to their bodies, hearts, and minds. From the days of knights and their ladies, thyme has been associated with courage—it can also be used as a thorough cleansing agent that is beneficial particularly when seasonal threats are high.

Men can use thyme as a reminder of courage and can choose to release what does not serve them. Traditionally, our society has dictated that men should be strong, exhibit no weak emotions and that crying is for girls. Because there are four root emotions (glad, sad, mad, afraid), most men opt unwittingly for the strong emotion—anger. It takes real courage to dig underneath that emotion to find that the root is fear or sadness.

Until you allow emotional honesty to occur on this level, you hold on to the reality you have created. Unless you are willing to revisit the real emotion behind the anger and connect to it, it is next to impossible to release it and let it go. Once you clear out what is not serving, you can powerfully restore your body, heart, and soul to experience and contribute on a much deeper level.

Let thyme remind you to release toxic emotions that frustrate and prevent close relationships with the people you love most. Choose to return to your authentic, caring, giving self, all the while realizing that courage is made of mastery of self.

Clove has a warm, spicy, woody aroma. It has powerful antioxidant properties, can be either stimulating or soothing depending on the situation, and promotes circulation and a healthy immune system.

As we maneuver our way through complicated interpersonal relationships, it's fairly common to experience pain, hurt, confusion, fear, and at times even abuse. Every person, at their core, wants to love and be loved. Sometimes, we just don't know how to go about it, so we put up a barricade around our hearts as a means of protection.

When diffused, we can draw strength intentionally from clove's warm and spicy aroma. We can remember that we have the responsibility to train others how we want to be treated. We can let it support us as we decide what it is we want and what we will accept. Each of us is priceless and worthy of love and happiness. All we have to do is create the path for getting there.

Clove's rich, fragrant aroma and powerful presence make it an ideal oil to use aromatically as we are physically and emotionally tuning into restoration. We are not victims of other people's choices. We are captains of our own souls, creating our own lives by intentional design. We are powerful beyond measure. Own your power, and choose an extraordinary life.

White fir is another incredibly rich oil that evokes feelings of stability, energy, and empowerment. It can be stimulating to the mind while helping the body to relax. Think of the qualities of a beautiful fir tree standing in the forest—it spices the air, sends roots deep beneath the earth, and extends a quiet calm that magnifies the peace found in nature. It absorbs carbon dioxide waste and metabolizes it into fresh oxygen. It shelters and protects numerous birds and animals. It has year-long life and presence. Trees are also symbolic of connecting us to our forebears, so they can remind us to strengthen our connection to family.

Another basic human need is our need for belonging. As we breathe in white fir, we can reaffirm our conviction that we *do* belong—that our presence on the planet this day, this time, is perfectly intentional. It is as it should be. We can use this time to ponder the fact that there are people who would not be the same without knowing us. Each of us has a purpose. Have we identified it?

Let the combined aromatic richness of white fir and clove help you let go of your to-do list or perfectionistic expectations and connect with your soul on a much deeper level. Get to know who you really are. You are timeless. Connecting with the perfect essence of who you really are will exponentially enhance the results of the restorative yoga sequence and prepare you to live your magnificence.

Sequence Instructions:

> **Props needed:** Yoga mat, two blocks, one strap, yoga bolster, eye pillow, and two yoga blankets
>
> **Practice preparation:** Find a quiet, comfortable space without distraction of technology. Carve out a time that no one might interrupt your opportunity to quiet your body, mind, and spirit. Keep an extra blanket on hand in case you get cold. Wear socks if you are cold natured. Once you have learned your place in each pose with the extent of props that make each position unique to supporting your frame, the time spent is meant to quiet the mind. This applies especially to the front of the brain that is always racing with worry, anxious feelings, and details of the to-do lists. Over time, with these poses, you will learn what tool(s) work better for you in your

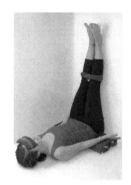

attempt to support your body and allow both body and mind to quiet Do not be disappointed in how your mind wanders—in yoga we call this "monkey-mind." Simply keep coming back to focusing on the tool you are using.

Here are some things to try:

1. Focus on the breath—this is very traditional and builds great awareness.
2. Focus on a pleasant memory; visualize the face of someone you love.
3. Use a mantra.
4. Pray.
5. Study a meditation beforehand and reflect on it or use a guided meditation.

Suggested length of time in each pose: 5–20 minutes. We've included very basic, acceptable, and effective poses in this section. You wouldn't necessarily want to practice all four of these restorative poses consecutively; just choosing one of them is adequate.

Insights about this sequence: Restorative poses are alignments designed to allow muscles to rest deeply. The use of props will allow adjustments to each individual frame so that the same experience of relief from tension on muscles, joints, and nerves will be common between all yogis.

Restorative Poses (Choose one or two to hold for 5–20 minutes each)
A. Viparita Karani—Legs up the Wall This pose takes the weight of the body off of the legs and the joints of the lower extremities. It is not important to be right up against the wall with the hips; two to three inches

Meditation brings wisdom; lack of meditation leaves ignorance. Know well what leads you forward and what holds you back, and choose the path that leads to wisdom.
—Buddha

away is traditional. Have a couple of blankets handy, a yoga strap, and it is optional to have sandbags and an eye pillow.

- To come into the pose, place a rectangular folded yoga blanket a couple of inches from the wall and sit sideways to the wall on the blanket. Lie down perpendicular to the wall on your yoga mat.
- Swing the legs up the wall and then make micro-adjustments in finding the distance from the wall that makes you comfortable.
- The folded blanket ends up under the pelvis to elevate the pelvis and allow a very gentle opening of the hips while supporting the lumbar curve. Seasoned yogis who are used to back-bending poses are more inclined to want two or more blankets or a small bolster to provide a deeper, passive back-bending effect.
- The strap should bind the legs together firmly, at the shins, close to the knee, and/or at the thighs. This helps to further relax the lower back.
- Sandbags are optional and two can be placed on top of the feet or one at each shoulder to add to the grounding effect.
- While resting arms with palms facing upward, smaller sandbags can be placed on the thumb-side of the palms to allow the front of the shoulders to open more by releasing tight pectoralis and anterior deltoid muscles.
- An eye pillow can be placed at the forehead to provide the aromatherapy. An eye pillow should not be placed on the eyes but on the brow, as the eyes are not meant to take pressure. The pillow also helps quiet the brain. Like shoulder stand, Viparita Karani will improve the health of the thyroid and condition the cardiovascular system because the heart now has to pump up to the legs.
- If the feet begin to tingle or get cold, draw the knees toward you, placing the feet ahead of the knees on the wall. Wait for the sensation to dissipate, and return the legs up for another minute or two. This is how you will build time in this pose as the body becomes conditioned to the alignment.

- Once this pose becomes familiar in your practice, you will recognize the quieting of the mind that then comes rather quickly. Try to stay 5–15 minutes.
- Once finished, plant the feet ahead of the knees on the wall, to bring the legs lower and to allow the cardiovascular system to readjust.
- Remove any props from underneath the pelvis to stretch the lower back more. Stay another minute here.
- Roll to your right and remain for a few breaths, then sit up in Sukhasana—Happy Pose—with the back supported against the wall for a minute to get your bearings and to reflect.

B. Supported Setu Bandha

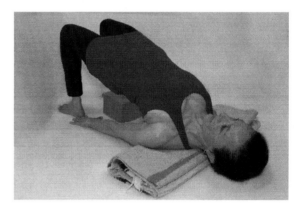

- Fold a yoga blanket or thick towel so that it is 8-to-12 inches wide. Place it across the yoga mat perpendicular to the length.
- Rest with your shoulders on the folded blanket and your head set lower on the mat.
- Plant your feet under your knees, hip width apart.
- Your head/neck may seem uncomfortable for just a few seconds until you are able to lift your hips and place the block—at first in a low position—under the hips against the flat part of the pelvis/sacrum. Here, the position of the neck should be level, parallel to the floor. If not, adjust with a small hand towel.
- Reach down lightly into the inner edges of the feet to keep the feet, ankles, knees, and hips from "turning out." This is a rest position, a passive hip flexor release, and a chest/shoulder opener. You can stay from 5-15 minutes.
- To come out of the pose, lift the hips, remove the block, gradually lower the body to the floor, slide down to allow the head to

rest on the blanket, rest here or roll to your side, and rest for a few breaths.

C. Legs in the Chair

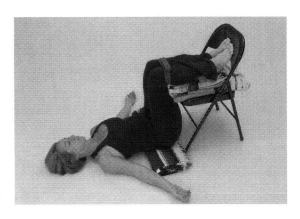

- This is an ideal position to release tension in the lower back.
- Rest on the floor—on your back—with the legs resting on the seat of a chair. Knees and hips must be at ninety degrees to make the support ideal. If the level of the seat of the chair is too low for the length of your legs, build up the height of the seat of the chair with extra blankets or a pillow.
- To support the lumbar spine, place a folded blanket under the pelvis still maintaining ninety degrees for the hips and knees.
- To enhance the lower-back release, bind the legs with a yoga strap at the thighs.
- Rest with arms thirty degrees away from your body, palms up, beside you on the floor, to invite the front of the shoulders to open.
- Use an eye pillow to help quiet the brain.
- To come out of the pose, release the strap at the legs, draw in the knees toward the chest, and place the feet on the edge of the chair with heels hanging off.
- Lift the hips, and remove the blanket if you had one there, and settle back down into this deeper lower-back release. Stay for 3–5 breaths.
- Working around the chair, roll to the side and rest for another 3–5 breaths so that the body is even and blood volume readjusts.
- Come up with Warrior I or Downward Facing Dog using the chair if you need it. Stand and lift the arms in Urdhva

You cannot always control what goes on outside. But you can always control what goes on inside.
—Mr. Yoga

201

Hastasana—Volcano pose. Lifting your gaze, take a deep breath, recognizing the quiet freedom in your body. Return the hands to Namaskarasana.

D. Savasana—Corpse Pose

This is a very simple rest position and generally opens the front body. This pose does not allow holding onto trauma, despair, or stress. Instead, it encourages "giving it away."

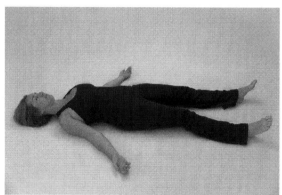

- A tight or compromised body may need some extra propping in this pose—a rolled up blanket or pillow under the knees to ease discomfort in the lower back, or a folded towel under the head to allow the neck to be neutral, parallel to the floor.
- Arms rest ideally out to the side, with palms up—thirty degrees away from the body to allow the front of the shoulders to open. Stay 5-20 minutes here.
- The following are ways to enhance the experience in all restorative poses:
  1. Cover with a blanket to keep the body warm, or wear socks and mittens.
  2. Use an eye pillow at the forehead to lift away worries. Consider aromatherapy by using a few drops of essential oils on the eye pillow.
  3. Use sandbags at the shoulders or hands to enhance shoulder opening

4. Use the rolled-up blanket under the upper thigh, instead, to open the hip flexors more, and traction the lumbar spine.

5. Align your pose with toes touching the wall ahead to create a "closed—circuit" which has a quieting effect for the central nervous system.

Yoga is a light, which once lit, will never dim. The better your practice, the brighter the flame.
—B. K. S. Iyengar

Restorative Sequence at-a-Glance

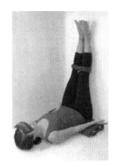

A. Viparita Karani /
Legs up the Wall

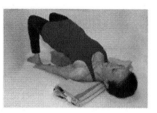

B. Supported
Setu Bandha

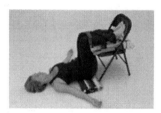

C. Legs in the
Chair

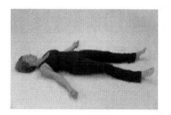

D. Corpse Pose

ABOUT THE AUTHORS

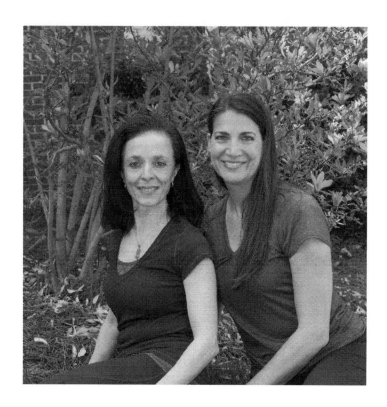

Mona Flynn

Mona Flynn, MS, RYT 500E, has spent more than 25 years studying and teaching in the wellness and fitness industries. She earned a B.S. in Exercise Physiology from Wake Forest University in 1987, and a Masters degree from James Madison University in 1989. She is a Yoga Alliance registered teacher since 2003, a member of the International Association of Yoga Therapists since 2005, founder of Lifefit Inc., and co-owner of the Institute of Integrated Yoga Therapy, a four level yoga teacher training school.

As a teacher, she applies knowledge from rehabilitative and alternative therapy practices into prevention methods, and incorporates the use of aromatherapy and essential oils for the benefit of her students. As a movement specialist, Mona combines knowledge and experience in applied anatomy, physiology, and biomechanics of movement. She emphasizes attention and care for safety and for recognizing individuals' needs, and educates and empowers students to prioritize self-care in their wellness practices.

Mona is a lifelong student of wellness, fitness and spirituality, and is always looking to improve her practice in continuing education and collaboration with others. She looks to lead her community in sharing knowledge and building relationships through public speaking, mentoring and community building efforts.

Outside of her profession, Mona spends her time gardening, sewing, and cooking, volunteering in her church, traveling and working with social justice organizations to help refugees resettle in the United States. She is a mother of two and lives in North Carolina with her husband.

Asti Atkinson
Asti Atkinson has been a wellness advocate and educator since 2010, and she has been using essential oils since 1998. Her natural wellness journey began when she became aware of essential oils. She became intrigued with the benefits of natural solutions for health and wellness and began to research and experience more. She discovered quickly that all essential oils are not created equal. She experienced firsthand the importance that sourcing, harvesting, extraction, and testing have on the purity and potency of the end product.

Her interests led to her passion for teaching others how to incorporate pure essential oils and other natural solutions into their lifestyles to assist with their emotional and physical wellbeing. Her passion also led to her interest in yoga in connection with the application of pure essential oils, both of which are ancient practices dating back thousands of years.

Asti has spoken at health and fitness events around the country. She has created and collaborated on wellness training programs and seminars—all designed to educate, empower, and inspire participants to incorporate natural solutions into their lifestyles. Asti also participates regularly in health and wellness training courses and seminars to increase her knowledge and expertise.

Asti lives in Utah with her husband and two sons. She loves to travel with her family and enjoys outdoor adventures including skiing, hiking, camping, and sailing.

ACKNOWLEDGMENTS

***Essential Yoga Practice* Book**

Foreword by Lillah Schwartz, E-RYT 500, author and Master Yoga Trainer

Cover Conceptualization by Matilda-Kirby Smith and Ariel Seymour

Cover by Ariel Seymour, Matilda-Kirby Smith, Marci Trakas, and Lauren McSwain

Social Media/Marketing by Lauren McSwain

Photo shoot at Greensboro Performing Arts:

http://www.greensboroperformingarts.com

Cassie Shintay, Photographer, models, and captures: cpshintay@gmail.com

Sam McClenaghan, Photographer and head shots: Sammac Photography,

http://sammacphotography.com

Nicola Young, Cecily Davis, Proofreading

Models:

Asti Atkinson

Benjamin Atkinson

Joshua Atkinson

Brooke Finch

Halah Flynn

John Flynn

Mona Flynn

Walker Flynn

Keely McKinney

Jennifer Merz

Jocelyn Mickey

Donna Phillips

Tom Phillips

Ariel Seymour

Alec Shepler

Leigha Shepler

Savannah Shepler

Bethany Staples
Dorle Webster
Emma Wheeler
Suzanne Vandergrift

www.essentialyogapractice.com and Social Media
Social Media/Marketing by Lauren McSwain
Sam McClenaghan, Photographer, headshots, http://sammacphotography.com

***Essential Yoga Practice* DVD**
Sam Hamlin, Videographer, Photographer, TEM Video: www.TEMVideo.com
Joy Hardy, Videographer, Photographer: TEM video
Ariel Seymour: Cover conceptualization and graphic design
Three sequences of this video were filmed at Stillwaters Retreat in Greensboro, North Carolina. http://stillwaters-retreat.com Owner, Donna Phillips

Yoga Models:
Asti Atkinson
Mona Flynn
Tracie Friddle
Helen Parrish
Dana Vaughn
Three sequences of this video were filmed at Christ United Methodist Church in Greensboro, North Carolina. http://www.christgreensboro.org.
Stage Skirt: Stage Decoration & Supplies, www.stagedec.com.

Yoga Models:
Hope Agresti
Asti Atkinson
Benjamin Atkinson
Joshua Atkinson
Brenda Bowman
Beth Burt
Drew Dodson
Mona Flynn

ACKNOWLEDGMENTS

Walker Flynn
Abby Gray
Lori Gray
Leslie Millsaps
Sophia Parker
Carmen Stanford
Klei Stanford

Special thanks to Nancy Pitkin, pianist, composer, sound healer, singer and song-writer for composing beautiful original music for the DVD. Songs included on the DVD are:
"Yellow Butterfly"
"Butterfly in Spring"
"Spirit Song"
"Lake of Dreams"
"Meditation for Ellen"
"Meditation on Jasper"
(All rights reserved)
For more information, visit www.nancypitkin.com

REFERENCES

Anderson, Sandra, and Rolf Lovik, PsyD. *Yoga, Mastering the Basics.* The Himilayan Institute, Honesdale, PA., 2000.

Ashafa A.O.T., D.S. Grierson and A.J. Afolayan, 2008. Effects of Drying Methods on the Chemical Composition of Essential Oil from *Felicia muricata* Leaves. *Asian Journal of Plant Sciences,* 7: 603-606.

Beattie, Melody. *Codependent No More: How to Stop Controlling Others and Start Caring for Yourself;* Hazelden; Center City, MN; 1992

Bellik, Yuva. "Total antioxidant activity and antimicrobial potency of the essential oil and oleoresin of *Zingiber officinale* Roscoe." *Asian Pac J Trop Dis.* 2014 Feb; 4(1): 40-44.

Bo, Pak. J. "Antioxidant Potential of Peel Essential Oils of Three Pakistani Citrus Species: Citrus Reticulata, Citrus Sinensis and Citrus Paradisii." *Pakistani Journal of Botany* 45.4 (2013): 1449-454. Accessed April 29, 2016. <http://www.pakbs.org/pjbot/PDFs/45(4)/48.pdf>.

Boyle, R., S. McLean, W. Foley, N. W. Davies, E. J. Peacock, and B. Moore. "Metabolites of dietary 1,8-cineole in the male koala (*Phascolarctos cinereus*)." *Comparative Biochemistry Physiology Part C Toxicology Pharmacology.* 129.4 (2001): 385–395. Accessed April 27, 2016. http://www.123helpme.com/view.asp?id=37810

Brokl, Michal, Marie-Laure Fauconnier, Celine Benini, Georges Lognay, Patrick Du Jardin, and Jean-Francois Focant. "Improvement of Ylang-Ylang Essential Oil Characterization by GC×GC-TOFMS." *Molecules.* 18.2 (2013): 1783-87. Accessed April 27, 2016. <http://www.mdpi.com/1420-3049/18/2/1783>.

Budig, Kathryn *The Women's Big Book of Yoga.* New York: Rodale Books, 2012), p.25.

Bullock, Grace; *"Yoga Can Change Your Brain: A Review of Research Provides Preliminary Evidence." Yoga U. Accessed April 10, 2016.* <https://www.yogauonline.com/yogau-wellness-blog/yoga-can-change-your-brain-review-research-provides-preliminary-evidence>.

Burney, Owen T., and Douglass F. Jacobs. "Terpene Production and Growth of Three Pacific Northwest Conifers in Response to Simulated Browse and Nutrient Availability." *Trees* 26.4 (2012): 1331-42. doi: 10.1007/s00468-012-0709-4, 23.

Carvalho Filho, Jose Luiz S. "Influence of the Harvesting Time, Temperature and Drying Period on Basil (*Ocimum Basilicum L.*) Essential Oil."*Www.scielo.br.* Revista Brasileira De Farmacognosia, 16.1 (2006):24-30. Accessed April 26, 2016. <https://dx.doi.org/10.1590/S0102-695X2006000100007>.

Chegini, I. Nezamivand. "Study the Nitrogen Rate Effect on Sweet Basil Phenological Stages and Physiological Indices under Different Plant Densities and Patterns." International Journal of Science and Advanced Technology 2.4 (2012): 25–33. Accessed April 26, 2016. <http://www.academia.edu/9787180/Study_the_Nitrogen_Rate_Effect_on_Sweet_Basil_Phenological_Stages_and_Physiological_Indices_under_Different_Plant_densities_and_Patterns_The_highest_seed_yield_obtained_in_N>.

Chien, L. W., S. L. Cheng, and C. F. Liu. "The Effect of Lavender Aromatherapy on Autonomic Nervous System in Midlife Women with Insomia." Evidence Based Complementary Alternative Medicine. (2011). doi: 10.1155/2012/740813.

Desikachar, T. K. V.; *The Heart of Yoga.* Rochester, VT: Inner Traditions International, 1995.

Diaz-Chavez, Maria L., Jessie Moniodis, Lufiani L. Madilao, Sharon Jancsik, Christopher I. Keeling, Elizabeth L. Barbour, Emilio L. Ghisalberti, Julie A. Plummer, Christopher G. Jones, Jörg Bohlmann. "Biosynthesis of Sandalwood Oil: *Santalum Album* CYP76F Cytochromes P450 Produce Santalols and Bergamotol." *PLoS One* 8.9 (2013). Accessed April 27, 2016. <http://dx.doi.org/10.1371/journal.pone.0075053>.

Dornelas, Marcelo Carnier. "A Genomic Approach to Characterization of the *Citrus* Terpene Synthase Gene Family." *Genetics and Molecular Biology* 30.3 (2007): 832–840. Accessed April 27, 2016. <https://www.researchgate.net/publication/228630111_A_ genomic_approach_to_characterization_of_the_Citrus_terpene_synthase_gene_ family>.

Edwards, Alan. "Insular Cortex Mediates Increased Pain Tolerance in Yoga Practitioners." Cerebreal Cortex 24 (2014): 2732–40. doi: 10.1093/cercor/bht124.

Emotions & Essential Oils: A Modern Resource for Healing Emotional Reference Guide. 3rd edition. Alpine, UT: Enlighten Alternative Healing, LLC, 2014.

Eppel, Elisa, Jennifer Daubenmier, Judith Moskowitz, Susan Folkman, Elizabeth Blackburn. "Can Meditation Slow Rate of Cellular Aging? Cognitive Stress, Mindfulness, and Telomeres." *Annals of the New York Academy of Sciences* 1172 (2009): 34–53. doi: 10.1111/j.1749-6632.2009.04414.x.

Fathi, E., and F. Sefidkon. "Influence of Drying and Extraction Methods on Yield and Chemical Composition of the Essential Oil of Eucalyptus sargentii." *Journal of Agricultural Science and Technology* 14 (2012):1035–42.

Filippi, Jean-Jacques, Emilie Belhassen, Nicolas Baldovini, Hugues Brevard, and Uwe J. Meierhenrich. "Qualitative and Quantitative Analysis of Vetiver Essential Oils by Comprehensive Two-dimensional Gas Chromatography and Comprehensive Two-dimensional Chromatography/mass Spectrometry." *Journal of Chromatography A* 1288 (2013): 127–48. Accessed April 28, 2016. doi: 10.1016/j.chroma.2013.03.002.

Frisch, Ashley J., and Karin E. Ulstru. "The Effects of Clove Oil on Coral: An Experimental Evaluation Using *Pocillopora Damicornis* (Linnaeus)." *Journal Experimental Marine Biology and Ecology* 345.2 (2007): 101–09. Accessed April 28, 2016. doi: 10.1016/j. jembe.2007.02.004.

Garber, Carol Ewing, Bryan Blissmer, Michael R. Deschenes, Barry A. Franklin, Michael J. Lamonte, I-Min Lee, David C. Nieman, and David P. Swain. "Quantity and Quality of Exercise for Developing and Maintaining Cardiorespiratory, Musculoskeletal, and Neuromotor Fitness in Apparently Healthy Adults: Guidance for Prescribing Exercise." American College of Sports Medicine Position Stand. *Medicine and Science in Sports and Exercise* 43.7 (2011):1334–59. Accessed April 10, 2016. doi: 10.1249/ MSS.0b013e318213fefb.

Gouyon, P. H., Ph. Vernet, J. L. Guillerm, and G. Valdeyron. "Polymorphisms and Environment:the Adaptive Value of the Oilpolymorphisms in Thymus Vulgaris L." *Heredity* 57.1 (1986): 59–66. Accessed April 28, 2016. www.researchgate.net.

Hay, Louise. *You Can Heal Your Life.* New York: Hay House, 2004.

Heagberg, Kat. "New Study Highlights Yoga's Cardiovascular Benefits." *Yoga International.* Last modified February 13, 2015. Accessed April 10, 2016. <https://yogainternational. com/article/view/new-study-highlights-yogas-cardiovascular-benefits>

Heagberg, Kat. "This is Your Brain on Yoga." *Yoga International.* Last modified January 15, 2014. Accessed April 20, 2016. <https://yogainternational.com/article/view/ this-is-your-brain-on-yoga>

Garber CE, Blissmer B, Deschenes MR, Franklin BA, Lamonte MJ, Lee IM, Nieman DC, Swain DP; http://www.ncbi.nlm.nih.gov/pubmed/21694556; American College of Sports Medicine; n.d; April 10, 2016

Hori, Etsuro, Hideo Shojaku, Naoto Watanabe, Yasuhiro Kawasaki, Michio Suzuk, Mariana F. P. de Araujo, Yoshinao Nagashima, Yukihiro Yada, Taketoshi Ono, and Hisao Nishijo. "Effects of Direct Cedrol Inhalation into the Lower Airway on Brain Hemodynamics in Totally Laryngectomized Subjects." *Autonomic Neuroscience* 168.1– 2 (2012): 88–92. Accessed April 28, 3016. doi:10.1016/j.autneu.2012.01.010

Iyengar, Geeta. *Yoga: A Gem for Women.* New York: Timeless Books, 2013.

Iyengar, B. K. S. *Yoga: The Path to Holistic Health.* London: Dorling Kindersley Limited, 2001.

Janaka, Jon. "Your Brain on Meditation." *Yoga International.* Last modified April 14, 2014. Accessed April 10, 2016. <https://yogainternational.com/article/view/your-brain-on-meditation>

Jin, Jingjing, Deepa Panicker, Qian Wang, Mi Jung Kim, Jun Liu, Jun-Lin Yin, Limsoon Wong, In-Cheol Jang, Nam-Hai Chua, and Rajani Sarojam. "Next Generation Sequencing Unravels the Biosynthetic Ability of Spearmint (*Mentha Spicata*) Peltate Glandular Trichomes through Comparative Transcriptomics." *BMC Plant Biology* 14 (2014): 292. Accessed April 28, 2016. doi: 10.1186/s12870-014-0292-5.

Johnson, Rebecca L., Steven Foster, Tieraona Low Dog, and David Kiefer. *National Geographic Guide to Medicinal Herbs: The World's Most Effective Healing Plants.* Washington, D.C.: National Geographic, 2012.

Jones, Christopher G., Christopher I. Keeling, Emilio L. Ghisalberti, Elizabeth L. Barbour, Julie A. Plummer, and Jörg Bohlmann. "Isolation of CDNAs and Functional Characterisation of Two Multi-product Terpene Synthase Enzymes from Sandalwood, *Santalum Album* L." *Archives Biochemistry Biophysics* 477.1 (2008): 121–30. Accessed April 28, 2016. doi:10.1016/j.abb.2008.05.008.

Jürgen, Leimner, Helga Marschall, Norbert Meier, and Peter Weyerstahl. "Italicene and Isoitalicene, Novel Ssquiterpene Hydrocarbons from Helichrysum Oil." *Chemistry Letters* 13.10 (1984): 1769–72. Accessed March 27, 2016. doi:10.1246/cl.1984.1769.

Kaur, Ramdesh. "7 Kundalini Mantras for 7 Seven Chakras." *Spirit Voyage.* Last modified September 24, 2014. Accessed April 10, 2016. <http://www.spiritvoyage.com/blog/index.php/7-kundalini-mantras-for-7-seven-chakras/?utm_source=Blog+Newsletter+July+22%2C+2014&utm_campaign=Newsletter+7-22-14&utm_medium=email>

Kondoh, Takashi, Shuori Yamada, Seiji Shioda, and Kunio Torii. "Olfactory Pathway in Response to Olfactory Stimulation in Rats Detected by Magnetic Resonance Imaging." *Chemical Senses* 30. supplement 1 (2005): i172–73, 2005. Accessed April 29, 2016. doi: 10.1093/chemse/bjh169.

Knasko, S. C. "Ambient Odor's Effect on Creativity, Mood and Perceived Health." *Chemical Senses* 17.1 (1992): 27–35. doi: 10.1093/chemse/17.1.27.Janaka, Jon. "Your Brain on Meditation." *Yoga International.* Last modified April 14, 2014. Accessed April 10, 2016. <https://yogainternational.com/article/view/your-brain-on-meditation>

Külheim, Carsten, Christopher G. Jones, Julie A. Plummer, Emilio L. Ghisalberti, Liz Barbour, and Jörg Bohlmann. "Foliar Application of Methyl Jasmonate Does Not Increase Terpenoid Accumulation, but Weakly Elicits Terpenoid Pathway Genes in Sandalwood (Santalum Album L.)." *Plant Biotechnology* 31 (2014): 585–91. Accessed April 29, 2016. doi: 10.5511/plantbiotechnology.14.1014a.

Kulisic, T., Ani Radonic, V. Katalinic, and Mladen Milos. "Use of Different Methods for Testing Antioxidative Activity of Oregano Essential Oil." *Food Chemistry* 85 (2004): 633–40. Accessed April 29, 2016. doi:10.1016/j.foodchem.2003.07.024.

Lal, R. K., Pankhuri Gupta, V. Gupta, Sougata Sarkar, and Smita Singh. "Genetic Variability and Character Associations in Vetiver (Vetiveria Zizanioides L. Nash)." *Industrial Crops and Products* 49 (2013): 273–77. Accessed April 29, 2016. doi:10.1016/j.indcrop.2013.05.005.

Lane, Alexander, Astrid Boecklemann, Grant Woronuk, and Soheil S Mahmoud. "A Genomics Resource for Investigating Regulation of Essential Oil Production in *Lavandula angustifolia.*" *Planta* 231.4 (2010): 835–45. Accessed April 29, 2016. doi: 10.1007/s00425-009-1090-4.

Lawless, Julia. *The Encyclopedia of Essential Oils: The Complete Guide to the Use of Aromatic Oils in Aromatherapy, Herbalism, Health, and Well Being.* San Francisco: Conan Press, 2002.

Li, Ying, Fabiano-Tixier, Anne-Silvie, and Chemat, Farid. *Essential Oils as Reagents in Green Chemistry.* 2014.

Lücker, Joost, Mazen K. el Tamer, Wlifried Schwab, Francel W. A. Verstappen, Linus H. W. van der Plas, Harro J. Bouwmeesster, and Harrie A. Verhoeven. "Monoterpene Biosynthesis in Lemon (*Citrus limon*)." *European Journal of Biochemistry* 269.13 (2002): 3160–71. Accessed April 29, 2016. <http://www.ncbi.nlm.nih.gov/pubmed/12084056>

Lukas, Brigitte, Rose Samuel, and Johannes Novak. "Oregano or Marjoram? The Enzyme γ-terpinene Synthase Affects Chemotype Formation in the Genus Origanum." *Israel Journal of Plant Science* 58 (2013): 211–20. Accessed April 29, 2016. doi:10.1560/IJPS.58.3-4.211

Maia, Marta Ferreira, and Sarah J. Moore. "Plant-based Insect Repellents: A Review of Their Efficacy, Development and Testing." *Malaria Journal* 10.Supplement 1 (2011):S11. Accessed April 29, 2016. doi: 10.1186/1475-2875-10-S1-S11.

Mazurek, Joanna. *Clearing Chakras with Essential Oils Helping You to Help Yourself.* Healthy Lifestyle with Essential Oils Book 1. Self published, 2014. Kindle edition.

Menon, A. Nirmala, K. P. Padmakumari, and Ananthasankaran Jayalekshmy. "Essential Oil Composition of Four Major Cultivars of Black Pepper (*Piper nigrum* L.)—IV." *Journal of Essential Oil Research* 17.2 (2005): 206–208. doi: 10.1080/10412905.2002.9699778.

Mindaryani, Aswati and Suprihastuti Sri Rahayu. "Essential Oil from Extraction and Steam Distillation of Ocimum Basillicum." *Proceedings of the World Congress on Engineering and Computer Science 2007* (n.d.): 90–94. Accessed April 27, 2016. <http://www.iaeng.org/publication/WCECS2007/WCECS2007_pp90-94.pdf>

Neumann, Janice. "Yoga May Benefit Heart Health as Much as Aerobics." *Reuters* December 26, 2014. Accessed April 10, 2016. <http://www.reuters.com/article/2014/12/26/us-health-yoga-cardio-trials-idUSKBN0K40Y520141226.>

Newberne, P., R. L. Smith, John Doull, J. I. Goodman, I. C. Munro, Phillip S. Portoghese, B. M. Wagner, C. S. Weil, L. A. Woods, T. B. Adams, C. D. Lucas, and Reena A. Ford. "The FEMA GRAS Assessment of *trans*-Anethole Used as a Flavouring Substance." *Food and Chemical Toxicology* 37.7 (1999): 789–811. doi: 10.1016/S0278-6915(99)00037-X.

Norrish, M. I. K., and K. L. Dwyer. "Preliminary Investigation of the Effect of Peppermint Oil on an Objective Measure of Daytime Sleepiness." *International Journal of Psychophysiology* 55.3 (2005): 291–298. doi: 10.3390/s110505469.

Ornish, Dean. *Dr. Dean Ornish's Program for Reversing Heart Disease: the Only System Scientifically Proven to Reverse Heart Disease without Drugs or Surgery.* New York: Random House, 1996.

Page, Martyn. *Human Body: An Illustrated Guide to Every Part of the Human Body and How It Works.* New York: Dorling Kindersley, 2001

Patora, Jolanta, Teresa Majda, Józef Góra, and Barbara Klimek. "Variability in the Content and Composition of Essential Oil from Lemon Balm (*Melissa Oficinalis* L.) Cultivated in Poland."*Acta Polonaie Pharmaceutica* Vol 60.5 (2003): 395–400. Accessed April 27, 2016. <https://www.researchgate.net/publication/7444393_Variability_in_the_content_and_composition_of_essential_oil_from_lemon_balm_Melissa_officinalis_L_cultivated_in_Poland>.

Peirce, Penney. *Frequency: The Power of Personal Vibration.* New York: Atria Books, 2009.

Raguso, Robert A. and Erin Pichersky. "New Perspectives in Pollination Biology: Floral Fragrances. A Day in the Life of a Linalool Molecule: Chemical Communication in a Plant-pollinator System. Part 1: Linalool Biosynthesis in Flowering Plants." *Plant Species Biology* 14.20 (1999): 95–120. doi: 10.1046/j.1442-1984.1999.00014.x.

Ramdani, Massaoud and Lograda, T. "Foliar Sesquiterpene Variations in Natural Populations of *Cupressus dupreziana* in Tassili N'Ajjer (Algeria)." *Asian Journal of Plant Sciences* 8.1 (2009): 59–63. doi: 10.3923/ajps.2009.59.63.

Rezaei Nejad, Abdolhossein and Ahmad. Ismaili. "Changes in Growth, Essential Oil Yield and Composition of Geranium (*Pelargonium graveolens* L.) as Affected by Growing Media." *Journal of the Science of Food and Agriculture* 94.5 (2014): 905–10. doi: 10.1002/jsfa.6334.

Rios-Estepa, Rigoberto, Glenn W. Turner, James M. Lee, Rodney B Croteau, and B. Markus Lange. "A Systems Biology Approach Identifies the Biochemical Mechanisms Regulating Monoterpenoid Essential Oil Composition in Peppermint." *Proceedings of the National Academy of Sciences of the United States of America* 105.8 (2008): 2818–23. doi: 10.1073/pnas.0712314105.

Saeio, Kiattisak, Wantida Chaiyana, and Siriporn Okonogi. "Antityrosinase and Antioxidant Activities of Essential Oils of Edible Thai Plants." *Drug Discoveries and Theraputics* 5.3 (2011): 144–49.

Satoh, Tamoko, and Yoshiaki Sugawara. "Effects on Humans Elicited by Inhaling the Fragrance of Essential Oils: Sensory Test, Multi-channel Thermometric Study and Forehead Surface Potential Wave Measurement on Basil and Peppermint." *Analytic Sciences* 19 (2003): 139–46. DOI: 10.2116/analsci.19.139.

Schnaubelt, Kurt. *The Healing Intelligence of Essential Oils: The Science of Advanced Aromatherapy.* Rochester, VT: Healing Arts Press, 2011.

Silva, Mira, and Shym Mehta. *Yoga: The Iyengar Way.* New York: Alfred A. Knopf, 2001.

Sparrowe, Linda, and Patricia Walden. *The Woman's Book of Yoga & Health.* Boston: Shambala Publications, 2002.

Takayama, Christiane, Felipe Meira De-Faria, Ana Cristina Alves De Almeida, Ricardo José Dunder, Luis Paulo Manzo, Eduardo Augusto Rabelo Socca, Leônia Batista, Marcos J. Salvador, Anderson Luis-Fierra, and Alba Regina Monteiro Souza-Brito. "Chemical Composition of *Rosmarinus Officinalis* Essential Oil and Antioxidant Action against Gastric Damage Induced by Absolute Ethanol in the Rat." *Asian Pacific Journal of Tropical Biomedicine,* 1/2016. Accessed April 27, 2016. doi: 10.1016/j. apjtb.2015.09.027.

Tanida, Mamoru, Akira Niijima, Jiao Shen, Takuo Nakamura, and Katsuya Nagai. "Olfactory Stimulation with Scent of Essential Oil of Grapefruit Affects Autonomic Neurotransmission and Blood Pressure." *Brain Research* 1058 (2005): 44–55.

Tosun, Murat, Sezai Ercisli, Memnune Sengul, Haan Ozer, Taskin Polat, and Erdogan Ozturk. "Antioxidant Properties and Total Phenolic Content of Eight *Salvia* Species from Turkey." *Biological Research* 42.2 (2009): 175–81. doi: /S0716-97602009000200005.

Turek, Claudia and Stintzing, Florian. "Stability of Essential Oils: A Review." *Comprehensive Reviews in Food Science and Food Safety* 12.1 (2013): 40–53. Accessed April 26, 2016. doi: 10.1111/1541-4337.12006.

Voo, Siau Sie, Howard D. Grimes, and B. Markus Lange. "Assessing the Biosynthetic Capabilities of Secretory Glands in Citrus Peel." *Plant Physiology* 159.1 (2012): 81–94. doi: 10.1104/pp.112.194233.

Williamson, Marianne. "Work." In *A Return to Love: Reflections on the Principles of A Course in Miracles*, 190. New York: HarperCollins, 1992.

Yuan, Jinhua, John R. Bucher, Thomas J. Goehl, Mike P. Dieter, and C. W. Jameson. "Quantitation of cinnamaldehyde and cinnamic acid in blood by HPLC." *Journal of Analytical Toxicology* 16.6 (1992): 359–62.

Yuma, Rubiya. *"Science on Meditation and Your Brain." Yoga International.* Accessed April 10, 2016. <https://yogainternational.com/article/view/science-on-meditation-and-your-brain>

Zarshenas, Mohammad M., Soliman Mohammadi Samani, Peyman Petramfar, and Mahmoodreza Moein. "Analysis of the Essential Oil Components from Different *Carum Copticum* L. Samples from Iran." *Pharmacognosy Research* 6.1 (2014): 62–66. Accessed April 27, 2016. doi: 10.4103/0974-8490.122920.

INDEX

38202845R00152